DID YOU KNOW . . .

Ginger can relieve both migraine headaches and the pain of rheumatoid arthritis . . .

Calcium and magnesium work wonders on menstrual cramps . . .

White willow will help with back pain, a condition that plagues up to 90% of Americans . . .

MSM, a dietary supplement, is revolutionizing the treatment of arthritis pain . . .

Magnet therapy may be your answer to relief from carpal tunnel syndrome, back pain, and more . . .

Colocynthis can stop painful colic in its tracks . . .

5-HTP, alone or with other natural pain killers, tackles fibromyalgia.

READ
NATURE'S PAINKILLERS
FOR MORE WAYS TO
FIGHT PAIN

ST. MARTIN'S PAPERBACKS TITLES
BY DEBORAH R. MITCHELL

Dictionary of Natural Healing

The Broccoli Sprouts Breakthrough

Nature's Painkillers

NATURE'S PAINKILLERS

DEBORAH R. MITCHELL

A Lynn Sonberg Book

St. Martin's Paperbacks

NATURE'S PAINKILLERS

Copyright © 2000 by Lynn Sonberg Book Associates.

All rights reserved. No part of this book may be used or reproduced in any manner whatsoever without written permission except in the case of brief quotations embodied in critical articles or reviews. For information address St. Martin's Press, 175 Fifth Avenue, New York, NY 10010.

ISBN: 0-312-97315-2

Printed in the United States of America

St. Martin's Paperbacks edition / April 2000

10 9 8 7 6 5 4 3 2 1

IMPORTANT NOTE:

This book is for informational purposes only. It is not intended to take the place of medical advice from a trained medical professional. Readers are advised to consult a physician or other qualified health professional regarding treatment of all of their health problems or before acting on any of the information or advice in this book.

This book is intended to provide selected information about supplements used for pain control. Research about natural methods of pain control is ongoing and subject to conflicting interpretations. As a result, there is no guarantee that what we know about this subject won't change with time.

The fact that a website or organization is listed in the book as a potential source of information does not mean that the author or publisher endorses any of the information they may provide or any of the recommendations they may make.

Contents

Introduction

When you're in pain, the first thing you need is safe, effective relief. The last thing you need are side effects that only compound your suffering. This book offers you the latest information about natural pain remedies. These treatments not only ease or eliminate your pain; they will do it naturally, without causing additional stress or damage to your body. *Nature's Painkillers* explains the different types of pain and the most effective herbal formulas, homeopathic remedies, and supplements that conquer it. The book also provides information on mind-body therapies and an energy therapy that is becoming increasingly popular—the use of magnets. These natural painkillers are easy to use, readily available, and virtually without side effects when compared with conventional treatments.

The *Merck Manual of Medical Information* defines pain as "an unpleasant sensation signaling that the body is damaged or threatened with an injury." Pain can be sharp or dull, fleeting or long term, isolated in one spot or feel as if it has invaded every inch of your body. Ask ten people to define and describe pain and you will likely get ten different answers, since no two cases of pain are alike, and they should not be treated with one-size-fits-all remedies, as conventional medicine often does.

Pain is universal yet individual; undeniably real yet no laboratory test can prove its existence or its severity. It is your friend (warns you when you touch a hot stove, for example) as well as an unwelcome intruder into your body and your life. And it invariably affects each and every person during his or her lifetime. Therefore, it is in your best interest to learn how to manage pain in the safest and most effective and most natural ways.

Great strides are being made in the field of pain and pain management. Although research traditionally has focused on developing new drugs to fight pain, interest in natural pain relievers is growing rapidly as more and more people search for safe, effective alternatives to conventional painkillers. Traditional drug treatments nearly always cause annoying or even debilitating side effects. And when you're in pain, the last thing you want—or need—is something that makes you feel worse.

This book offers usable, comprehensive information about more than 30 of the most effective natural pain relievers. Before you delve into the wealth of information about these remedies and learn how to incorporate them into your own life, it is important to understand the type of pain you are trying to eliminate or relieve. Chapter 1 answers such questions as:

What is pain? and What are the types of pain? In Chapter 2 you will read about conventional pain medications, how they could be causing you harm, and how natural pain relievers may be the alternative you are seeking.

Chapter 3 explains the most common painful conditions and then refers you to Chapters 4 and 5, where you get in-depth explanations about the appropriate natural pain relievers for those conditions.

Chapter 3 is followed by an easy reference chart that allows you to identify the most effective natural painkillers for the painful conditions for which you seek relief. Chapters 4 and 5 contain detailed information on natural painkillers from the fields of herbal medicine, homeopathy, and nutrition; mind-body medicine; and energy therapy. Each entry discusses the specific types of pain the remedy treats best, how the remedy works, the proof and reports behind the claims, how you can use the remedy for yourself, and any safety factors and other relevant information that can allow you to best utilize these methods. You will learn, for example:

- How to use ginger to relieve migraine headache and the pain of rheumatoid arthritis
- What experts and patients say about magnet therapy, an evolving energy treatment that has proven effective in treating all types of pain, from backache to menstrual cramps
- Why the Chinese swear by the painkilling ac-

tions of angelica root, corydalis, ligusticum, and other herbs
- The magic of magnesium in relieving migraine headache and PMS symptoms
- How a problem that plagues up to 90 percent of Americans—back pain—can be relieved or eliminated with white willow, arnica, rhus toxicodendron, and other gifts of Nature
- Convenient ways to incorporate more than 20 different natural painkillers into your everyday life

Natural pain relief is three easy steps away:

1. Find the condition you want to treat in Chapter 3, read about it, and find which remedies are recommended.
2. Turn to those remedies in Chapters 4 and 5 and read all about them, including how they work, how to take them, and any precautions you should know.
3. Read Chapter 6 on how to buy and use the pain remedy that you have chosen, then get that remedy (after talking with your healthcare provider, of course).

Pain may be a part of life, but it need not control your life. *Nature's Painkillers* helps you take back control of your pain and your life in a safe, effective, natural way.

CHAPTER ONE

Pain: What You Need to Know to Make It Go Away

Sharp. Dull. Stabbing. Throbbing. Piercing. Gnawing. Cutting. Annoying or debilitating, temporary or chronic, pain is a part of life. Be it from arthritic joints, a scraped knee, a broken bone, a paper cut, or a blinding migraine, it moves in and out of our lives, sometimes staying away for days or weeks, other times lingering or returning again and again. It's been called a friend and a gift because it warns us that something in the body needs to be attended to or healed, and that warning can literally save our lives. Yet, as Dr. Paul Brand and Philip Yancey say so aptly in the title of their book, pain is "the gift nobody wants."

On the surface, pain seems like a simple thing: It's when your body or mind (emotions), or both, hurt. But a migraine hurt is not like a bruised finger hurt; nor is a broken toe like the hurt of back pain. There are different types of pain with different causes and, it follows, different ways to treat these various kinds of hurt. In this chapter you will learn things about pain that will help you make it go away, beginning with two basic yet important questions:

- What is pain? A simple question with a not-so-simple answer.
- What are the various types and categories of pain?

What Is Pain?

Pain, according to the International Association for the Study of Pain, is "an unpleasant sensory and emotional experience normally associated with tissue damage or described in terms of such damage." A group of experts from the University of Western Ontario came up with a similar definition and expanded on it to say that "Pain is always subjective. Each individual learns the application of the word into experiences related to injury in early life . . . it is also always unpleasant and therefore also an emotional experience." These definitions tell you two things: Pain is physical, and pain is emotional. And because the answer to the simple question "What is pain?" involves both the body and mind, this definition also tells you that the answer is not simple.

Aristotle called pain "a passion of the soul," and indeed we cannot separate the physical from the emotional when it comes to pain. As you'll read later under "Types of Pain" and in Chapter 5, the mind—emotions, feelings, and thoughts—plays a huge role in the perception, management, and control of pain.

The answer to the question "What is pain?" is equally complex on a scientific level. Scientists can study pain subjectively by assigning intensity scales (how much it hurts on a scale of 1 to 10, with 10 being the most pain), yet pain itself cannot be seen or observed. When you say to someone, "That looks like it hurts" or "That looks painful," you cannot "see" the pain. Yet you may, in fact, actually feel the pain physically, even though you are not the one who has the injury, disease, or other tissue damage that is causing the physical pain. You have an emotional sense of the pain.

Given that pain has such a complex nature, perhaps the best way to answer the question is to explain how pain works. The pain cycle can be explained in three steps.

1. Pain receptors, which are found throughout the body, are stimulated by some type of event or incident (e.g., touching a hot stove, hitting your finger with a hammer, or having a tooth pulled). The receptors transmit the message of pain as electrical impulses along the nerves to the spinal cord.

2. The incoming pain messages arrive at the spinal cord and are sent along to the brain. At the same time, some messages may trigger a reflex response, if the situation is appropriate; for example, if you hit your thumb with a hammer, you immediately pull your hand away. In such

cases, once the pain signals reach the spinal cord, a reflex response signal is sent back to the site of the injury while the pain signals go on to the brain. You do not become consciously aware of the pain, however, until step 3, after the reflex action.

3. The brain processes the pain signal, even though you already have had (a split second earlier) a reflex response, and you feel the pain.

Step 3 is where the popular concept, "gate-control theory," can be explained. Ronald Melzack, Ph.D., and Patrick Wall, M.D., two pain research pioneers, proposed that thousands of nerve fibers converge at a series of "gates" where the brain and spinal cord meet. At those points, some pain signals get through and others may not, depending on the type of pain and the state of mind of the receiver of the pain. People have the ability to control the amount of pain that gets through the gates. This idea helps explain such phenomena as how people can use their mind to control pain (e.g., walking on hot coals), the success of acupuncture (stimulation from the needle crowds out pain signals), and other more ordinary occurrences such as relieving headache pain by practicing deep breathing.

To complicate matters, not all pain receptors and their associated nerve transmission pathways are the same. The pain receptors in your hand, for example, differ from those in your large intestine. If you cut your finger with a knife, you can identify the feeling (sharp) and precisely where the pain is occurring (an example of *localized pain*). A cut into your intestinal wall, however, would not generate a localized pain response. If a gas bubble were trapped in your intestines, however, you could feel a great deal of pain, yet the pain would be spread over the entire intestinal tract rather than in one precise spot (an example of *generalized pain*).

Different parts of the body have varying numbers of pain receptors, depending on each part's need to register pain. The eye, for example, is very vulnerable to injury and so it is about 1,000 times more sensitive to pain than the bottom of the foot. Pain receptors also respond to stimulation at different speeds. A painful stimulus to the skin, such as touching a hot iron, sends signals at a rate of 300 feet per second; pain signals from an internal organ move along at two feet per second.

Another factor that comes into play is people's ability to tolerate pain, which is based on personality, perspective, and the circumstances under which pain occurs. One woman with menstrual cramps may have the attitude that nothing will stop her as she works, hikes, and barrels through her day. Another woman may want to pamper herself, relax on the couch all day, and clutch a hot water bottle. A positive attitude and participation in activities that divert attention away from pain are ways the mind can manage and control pain, while feeling like a victim and focusing on the pain as a negative thing can make it worse. The pain signals for both women may be similar, yet how they perceive the pain differs. Likewise, a runner may twist his or her ankle during a race and go on to finish it without noticing the pain until later when the excitement and the flow of endorphins (discussed below) have gone.

What Role Does Inflammation Play in Pain?

Pain and inflammation typically go hand in hand. Inflammation is an accumulation of fluids in the injured or affected area that transports cells from the immune system to the injured area. This is a good response, because the fluids destroy or prevent toxins and damaged tissue from accumulating at the site. The immune system cells attack free radical cells, highly active molecules that destroy healthy cells and contribute to pain. (One way free radicals can cause pain is through the destruction of healthy cartilage cells, which contributes to the pain of osteoarthritis.) At the same time, cells in the area of the tissue damage release chemicals that irritate the nerves. These nerves send pain signals to the spinal cord and brain. Some of the chemicals trigger muscle spasms, which protect the injured area from movement but which also contribute to pain. The blood vessels also respond by growing narrower and reducing the amount of bleeding. Thus inflammation is beneficial, but it also produces more pain as it presses on nerves and tissue in the affected area of the body.

Fortunately, inflammation is short-lived for many people. As the damaged tissue heals and the toxins are eliminated, the pain and inflammation subside. For people with chronic pain that involves inflammation, however, the inflammation process has gone haywire. Rheumatoid arthritis, osteoarthritis, interstitial cystitis, and lupus are examples of conditions in which inflammation has become unregulated.

Types of Pain

Pain can be either acute or chronic. *Acute* pain comes on suddenly, can be mild to severe, has an identifiable cause, and usually doesn't last very long. The pain may arise from an injury, such as a burn or cut; or it may be an occasional pain, such as a tension headache or an earache. If the pain is severe, as it can be with an attack of appendicitis or labor pains, it may be accompanied by dilated pupils, sweating, and an increase in heart rate, blood pressure, or breathing rate.

Chronic pain usually is described as pain that: lasts for weeks or longer, keeps returning over a period of months or years, persists for more than one month beyond the normal course of an injury or disease, or is associated with a long-term disease such as diabetes, cancer, or AIDS. Often chronic pain is accompanied by insomnia, or troubled sleep, constipation, decreased appetite, weight loss, depression, and loss of libido.

Chronic pain occurs when the body's response to pain becomes impaired or goes awry, or when the pain associated with a specific medical condition or disease becomes prolonged or persistent. Examples include arthritis, fibromyalgia, migraine, back pain, and carpal tunnel syndrome.

Doctors and scientists still have much to learn and understand about chronic pain. Dr. Wall and Dr. Melzack, whose theories on pain originally appeared in *Science* in 1965, explain that chronic pain is a complicated process, much more so than acute pain, and that we still do not know exactly why it develops. In cases of acute pain, treatment and time are the healers, and the pain disappears eventually. With chronic pain, the initial trigger may be the same as in acute pain—a fall, a tooth extraction, a stomach virus, or a pain in the back or head that appears for no apparent reason. Yet after treatment and a reasonable amount of time, the pain doesn't go away, or it gets worse, or it recurs again and again.

Research indicates that the pain may persist because some of the damaged nerves do not heal properly, so they continue to send pain messages even though there is no injury. If the spinal cord keeps receiving high levels of pain signals, eventually the cord can lose its ability to regulate the messages, and the result is chronic pain. If we consider the gate-control theory, chronic pain may be an example of the gates staying open, allowing pain signals to keep going to the brain, unregulated and out of control.

Categories of Pain

Pain is the most common symptom of disease, yet you do not need to have a disease in order to have pain. Indeed, two of the most common types of pain— backache and headache—are usually not associated with a disease but with lifestyle.

Pain can be categorized in several different ways, based on where or how the pain originates, how it is manifested, or if it is associated with a disease or condition. The U.S. Department of Health and Human Services (HHS) has named the following major categories of chronic pain: arthritic, back (lower), cancer, headache, neurogenic (damaged nerves), and psychogenic (pain of unknown cause). A brief list of different categories of pain follows; it incorporates the HHS list as well as those of other institutions involved in the study and treatment of pain. Details about each of these categories and the painful conditions within them follow in Chapter 3:

- Arthritis pain
- Childhood disorders
- Gynecological and menstrual pain
- Headache and migraine
- Muscle, sports, and overuse-related pain
- Neurological pain
- Postsurgical pain
- Other painful conditions

Other Painful Conditions

Medical conditions also discussed in Chapter 3 that do not fit into the categories just mentioned include: cystitis, gallbladder disorders, hemorrhoids, irritable bowel syndrome, liver disorders, sinusitis, temporomandibular joint syndrome (TMJ), and ulcers.

Now that you have an idea of how complex pain can be, you can better appreciate why often it is difficult to eliminate and why there are so many different pain medications on the market. The next chapter takes a close look at conventional pain relievers and the problems they can cause and then introduces you to the world of nature's painkillers.

CHAPTER TWO

Problems with Conventional Painkillers

Aspirin. Ibuprofen. Codeine. Morphine. Many people are familiar with these painkillers, especially the first two, which are found in medicine cabinets in many homes in the United States. Yet despite the widespread use of conventional painkillers, one of their main problems is that they fail to take care of the cause of the pain. That's because they work by suppressing awareness of the pain rather than addressing the *cause* of the pain. Thus the pain is still there, beneath the mask of the painkiller you took. Once the painkiller wears off, you will need another dose, and another. Until the body takes care of the pain's source, you learn to live with the pain, or you become dependent upon painkillers.

In this chapter you will learn about conventional painkillers and treatments—including over-the-counter and prescription drugs and surgery—what they can and cannot do, and their side effects. You also will be introduced to natural painkillers and how they work, and how and when you can use conventional and natural pain relievers together.

Over-the-Counter Pain Relief

Painkillers, or analgesics, make up 25 percent of the over-the-counter drug market. Each year Americans take more than 50 billion over-the-counter (OTC) pain relief products. Four types of OTC analgesics are available: aspirin, ibuprofen, naproxen, and acetaminophen. Aspirin has been in use in one form or another since ancient times, when Hippocrates used a derivative of willow bark to relieve pain. Aspirin became available in tablet form in 1899, and now Americans take about 29 billion of those tablets a year. Ibuprofen broke onto the pain management scene and joined aspirin as members of a classification of drugs called nonsteroidal anti-inflammatory drugs, or NSAIDs; they are discussed together next. Naproxen, another NSAID, is similar in structure and effect to ibuprofen. Acetaminophen, which currently outsells aspirin for relief of pain, does not reduce inflammation and is considered to be safer by some experts, although this claim is disputed by others.

Despite the fact that OTC pain relievers carry warning labels, Americans know surprisingly little about the drugs they take. According to a survey conducted by the American Pharmaceutical Association, 47 percent of adults don't always read the labels on their medications, less than 40 percent ask a pharmacist about the drugs, 74 percent do not associate stomach bleeding or discomfort with aspirin use, and 43 percent are not aware that there are potential risks from taking OTC drugs and prescription medications at the same time. (For more details, see *Dangerous Drug Interactions* by Teresa and Joe Graedon, in the Bibliography.)

NSAIDs

The main attraction of NSAIDs in the treatment of pain is that they reduce inflammation, which they do by having an effect on hormonelike substances called prostaglandins. Prostaglandins are released to the body site when and where cells are damaged or stimulated. Once they arrive, prostaglandins can play several roles, depending on their type. Some cause inflammation while others increase the awareness of pain or promote the clotting of blood. Aspirin and other NSAIDs interfere with the prostaglandin production and so suppress inflammation and awareness of pain.

Taking something that suppresses inflammation and your awareness of pain sounds like a great deal—at first. But you may pay a big price for that temporary relief in the form of bothersome or even dangerous side effects, including bleeding of the stomach lining and ulcers. (See Table 2.1.) The reason NSAIDs cause stomach and intestinal disorders is that they block the activity of two enzymes, cyclooxygenase-1 and cyclooxygenase-2 (COX-1 and COX-2). COX-1 is responsible for pain and inflammation, so blocking its effects is good. However, NSAIDs also block COX-2, which suppresses the prostaglandins that protect the stomach and kidneys. Thus when you take NSAIDs, you prevent prostaglandins from doing their "good work" as well. Anyone with kidney disease, cirrhosis, or a diagnosis of heart failure who takes NSAIDs must take additional precautions. These individuals may experience kidney toxicity after taking the drugs for only a few days, and the consequences can be fatal.

People who think that nonaspirin NSAIDs are easier on the stomach than aspirin should read the warning labels. After a 1986 study found that people older than 60 who took nonaspirin NSAIDs were three times as likely as nonusers to require hospitalization because of bleeding ulcers, the Food and Drug Administration (FDA) required new warnings on these drugs.

Some aspirin and other NSAIDs are buffered, or coated, with calcium carbonate, magnesium oxide, or other antacids to help prevent stomach upset or heartburn. Buffering does not change the fact that NSAIDs prevent prostaglandins from doing their "good work," so stomach damage is still possible. In addition, buffered drugs can take twice as long to provide pain relief as plain aspirin, which prompts some people to become frustrated and to take higher doses than they should.

Acetaminophen

Millions of people turn to acetaminophen (e.g., Tylenol) as an alternative over-the-counter analgesic because it is gentler on the stomach lining than NSAIDs. However, acetaminophen can cause liver damage when taken in large doses for a prolonged period. In 1995 the *New England Journal of Medicine* reported that people who take acetaminophen regularly have an increased risk of advanced kidney disease.

Acetaminophen can be especially dangerous for children who accidentally overdose on the drug. As few as 10 Extra-strength Tylenol can be fatal to a child, while a comparable amount of aspirin generally will not.

No one is sure exactly how acetaminophen works, but a popular theory is that it acts on the nerve endings to mask pain. Acetaminophen is comparable to aspirin when it comes to relieving mild to moderate pain but less effective in relieving muscle sprains and strains.

NSAIDs

Common NSAIDs on the market:
Aspirin, choline magnesium trisalicylate, diclofenac, diflunisal, fenoprofen, flurbiprofen, ibuprofen (Motril, Advil), indomethacin (Indocin), ketoprofen, meclofenamate, nabumetone, naproxen (Aleve, Naprosyn), oxaprozin, phenyl-

butazone, piroxicam (Feldene), salsalate, sulindac (Clinoril), tolmetin

Prescription Analgesics: COX-2 Inhibitors

The first of a new class of pain relief drugs was introduced to the prescription market on December 31, 1998. Celebrex (generic name, celecoxib) made its debut in the new category, called COX-2 inhibitors, which rival NSAIDs in that they do not cause the gastrointestinal problems associated with NSAID use. Another trade brand, Vioxx (generic name, rofecoxib), was approved by the FDA on May 20, 1999. Unlike NSAIDs, COX-2 inhibitors do not block the enzyme that protects the stomach and kidneys, COX-1, while they inhibit the action of COX-2 enzymes.

The FDA approved celecoxib for the treatment of osteoarthritis and rheumatoid arthritis only, not for general pain management. People with liver problems, a diagnosis of heart failure, preexisting asthma, water retention, or who are taking lithium or fluconazole (Diflucan) should not take celecoxib without first consulting their physician.

Prescription Analgesics: Opioids

All opioid analgesics are chemically related to morphine and act directly on the nervous system. Although very effective in masking pain, opioid analgesics also have significant side effects, including chemical dependence and severe withdrawal symptoms if the drugs are not stopped correctly. The degree of physical dependence and the length of time it takes to develop vary, depending on the drug taken. Generally, however, people who take opioids become physically dependent over time.

Side effects from normal use include constipation, drowsiness, vomiting, and nausea. High doses can cause difficulty breathing and coma. Opioid analgesics include codeine, hydromorphone, levorphanol, morphine, meperidine, methadone, oxymorphone, oxycodone, pentazocine, propoxyphene.

TABLE 2.1
OTC Pain Relievers
Products Containing Aspirin

With prolonged use, any of these products can cause irritation and/or bleeding of the gastrointestinal tract, ringing in the ears, allergic reactions in people who are sensitive to aspirin, Reye's syndrome in children and teenagers (a disease that can cause seizures, brain damage, and death), and complications of labor in pregnant women. Aspirin should be avoided by anyone who has ulcers, asthma (it can trigger an attack), or liver or kidney disease.

Alka-Seltzer with aspirin
Ascriptin A/D
Aspergum
Aspirin

Bayer: Genuine Bayer Aspirin tablets, Maximum Bayer Aspirin tablets, Children's Aspirin, 8-Hour Bayer Timed-Release caplets

Bufferin and Bufferin Extra Strength

Ecotrin tablets and Ecotrin Maximum Strength tablets

Empirin

Halfprin 81

St. Joseph's Adult Chewable Aspirin

Products Containing Ibuprofen (I), Ketoprofen (K), or Naproxen (N)

Any of these nonaspirin products can cause irritation of the digestive tract and allergic reactions in sensitive individuals, Prolonged use can cause ulcers and kidney damage in the elderly and other susceptible people.

Actron (K)

Advil (I)

Aleve (N)

Bayer Select Pain Relief Formula (I)

Excedrin IB (I)

Haltran (I)

Ibuprofen (I)

Ibuprin (I)

Medipren (I)

Midol IB (I)

Motrin IB (I)

Nuprin (I)

Orudis KT (K)

Pamprin-IB (I)
Trendar (I)

Products Containing Acetaminophen

Any of these products can cause kidney damage with prolonged use, liver damage when taken at high doses over a prolonged period of time, or allergic reactions in sensitive individuals. They should not be taken on an empty stomach or with alcohol.

Anacin-3, Anacin-3 Children's, Aspirin Free Anacin Maximum Strength

Arthritis Pain Formula Aspirin Free

Datril Extra Strength

Liquiprin Elixir

Panadol, Junior Strength Panadol

St. Joseph Aspirin-Free Fever Reducer for Children

Tempra

Tylenol caplets, Tylenol Children's, Tylenol Junior Strength, Tylenol Extra Strength

Surgery as Pain Reliever

Surgery is the most radical and invasive way to manage pain and should be considered only after all other avenues have been explored. For many people who suffer with intractable pain, surgery may seem like the only solution. For those with chronic back pain, surgery may seem like a silver bullet. More than

250,000 back surgeries are performed each year in the United States to remove herniated disks, and tens of thousands of other back operations are done for other painful conditions. Yet many of these surgeries could be avoided, and unfortunately even when they are performed oftentimes the pain is not eliminated.

For example, a procedure called a diskectomy, in which people with a herniated disk (also called a slipped disk) have part of the disk removed from the spine, has a good (90 to 95 percent) success rate initially. Within 10 years, recurring herniation and scarring bring the percentage down to 70 percent or less. A more advanced form of diskectomy, called microdiskectomy, allows surgeons to make a smaller incision and to use a high-powered microscope to view the surgical area. Relief of back pain occurs in less than 90 percent of patients, and many need an additional operation because the doctors often need to recover disk fragments not seen during the original surgery. A similar problem occurs with percutaneous diskectomy, in which the disk fragments are removed with suction through a tiny incision.

Cutting the nerves that send pain signals from the body to the brain is another surgical alternative. This method is used for some individuals who have facet-joint pain (joint in the spine where two adjacent vertebrae meet) and occasionally for people with trigeminal neuralgia. (See "Neuralgia" in Chapter 3.) Even this step, however, may not eliminate the pain.

How Natural Painkillers Work

~~~⌒~~~

While conventional painkillers suppress the awareness of pain, natural painkillers get to the heart of the matter—the cause of the pain. You know that pain produces inflammation, and inflamed tissues press on nerves, which causes more pain. Then the free radicals converge on the injured scene, bringing on more pain.

Natural pain relievers go to work on the inflammation and the free radicals. Depending on the remedy you choose, it may reduce fluid levels at the hurting site (e.g., turmeric, boswellia), reduce the excitability of nerve cells (e.g., magnesium), or reduce inflammation (e.g., hypericum, willow bark).

Using Natural Painkillers and Conventional Methods

~~~⌒~~~

One of the advantages of natural pain relievers is that in most cases, they can be used safely and effectively with conventional methods, if you choose to do so. (*NOTE: Consult with your physician before you start taking any natural pain relievers or beginning any natural therapies, especially if you are currently taking conventional medications.*) In many cases, people can significantly reduce or even eliminate their need for conventional painkillers once they start with natural methods. Because many prescription painkillers can cause withdrawal symptoms, it is important for you to work with your physician to slowly reduce your drug usage.

Unlike conventional medications, which cause side effects and require caution when taking more than one at a time, Nature's painkillers work in harmony with the body and with most other substances, natural and conventional. In fact, it is not unusual to combine herbs to make a tonic, to mix two or more homeopathic remedies together for specific ailments, or to take nutritional supplements while you are taking a course of herbal or homeopathic remedies. Nearly all Chinese herbal remedies are a combination of herbs especially chosen to work in balance with each other and with the body. Natural pain relief substances plus mind-body therapy is an ideal pairing because it allows you to integrate physical and mental control over your pain in a safe manner.

One area that demonstrates the complementary relationship between natural and conventional medicine is in the relief of postsurgical pain and inflammation. Studies show that taking homeopathic remedies before and immediately after a surgical procedure can reduce pain and the amount of narcotic analgesics needed for pain control, increase the body's ability to heal, and reduce bruising. Homeopathic remedies can be taken sublingually (under the tongue) right before you go into the operating room without fear of nausea or vomiting. **Arnica** and **hypericum**, two remedies commonly used for this purpose, are discussed in detail in Chapter 4.

Use of herbal remedies for arthritis pain is becoming more and more common as people are concerned about the adverse effects associated with conventional arthritis medications. The addition of natural remedies such as boswellia, bromelain, and ginger to a treatment plan that includes acetaminophen or opioids can quickly result in a reduction or even eventual withdrawal of the conventional drugs.

Mind-body and energy therapies also are excellent complements to conventional medical practices. Many patients who make the commitment to use mind-body or energy methods to control or eliminate their pain do so because they don't like the feeling of helplessness and lack of control that comes from depending on medications. Methods such as biofeedback, hypnosis, meditation, visualization, and magnetic therapy—all discussed at length in this book—put pain control into the hands of the person in pain rather than in the hands of a physician, pharmacist, or therapist. Again, however, if you are taking prescription medication for pain and are using mind-body or energy techniques, let your healthcare provider know so he can advise you on whether you can withdraw from your medication and do so safely.

Understanding pain is essential if you want to learn to control and perhaps eliminate it. Now that you know a bit about what pain is and how it works, let's explore some of life's most painful conditions and the natural pain relievers that may be most effective against them.

CHAPTER THREE

Painful Conditions and How to Get Relief

Pain is an equal opportunity annoyer: It doesn't care about color, religion, education, ethnic background, economic class, or sex. Pain, like a smile and laughter, also transcends the language barrier. You don't need to speak the language of another person if you are in pain: Your face and your actions will convey the message.

Natural, safe, nonpharmaceutical remedies are available. Do you know what they are and which types of pain they can treat effectively? In this chapter you will read about the most common painful conditions, the types of pain they cause, and which natural pain remedies may be most effective in reducing or eliminating the pain. Find the conditions for which you are seeking pain relief. After you have read the entry, refer to the remedies that are recommended, which are explained in depth in Chapters 4 and 5. *Note:* The mind-body and energy therapies suggested for specific conditions are those that have been discussed the most in the literature. This does not mean these methods would not work for other painful ailments. You are encouraged to consider these alternative therapies for any pain you may have, because the mind itself is the only limit on its power.

Warning: Because the belladonna plant is poisonous (though the homeopathic remedy is not), use only the homeopathic form of belladonna and follow your health-care provider's instructions for use.

Arthritis Pain

More than 100 different conditions are classified under the category "arthritis," a general term that refers to inflammation of the joints. Approximately 15 percent of Americans suffer from some form of arthritis. The most common forms are discussed below.

Osteoarthritis
Approximately 40 million Americans suffer with this type of arthritis, which results from wear and tear on the joints. Osteoarthritis, which is also known as degenerative joint disease, is characterized by joint pain and stiffness caused by a degeneration of the joint cartilage and the adjacent bone. The joints most often affected are those in the fingers, the base of the thumbs, neck, lower back, big toes, hips, and knees. As the damage to the joints worsens, mobility decreases.

Osteoarthritis can be primary or secondary. Primary osteoarthritis occurs without any apparent preexisting abnormalities. Scientists believe the process of aging and its wear and tear on the joints has a cumulative destructive effect on the collagen matrix, which supports the cartilage. Secondary osteoarthritis develops because of a predisposing situation, such as a preexisting abnormality in the bone or cartilage, trauma (which may include a fracture or surgery), or the presence of another inflammatory joint disease (e.g., gout, rheumatoid arthritis).

An interesting feature of osteoarthritis is that the degree of damage to the cartilage and joints does not necessarily correlate with the level of pain people experience. Physicians find that about 40 percent of patients with X-ray evidence of severe osteoarthritis have little or no pain, yet some people with joints that appear normal have terrible pain.

Natural Remedies: Arnica, belladonna, boswellia, bromelain, calcarea carbonica, calcarea phosphorica, cayenne (capsaicin), Chinese herbs, devil's claw, ginger, glucosamine, marijuana, MSM, rhus toxicodendron, white willow, magnet therapy, guided imagery.

Rheumatoid Arthritis and Similar Diseases

An estimated 2 million people are afflicted with rheumatoid arthritis, an intractable and painful form of arthritis that affects the entire body but is most evident in the joints. Rheumatoid arthritis is characterized by painful swelling, inflammation, and stiffness in the limbs, wrists, and fingers. Often the involved joints are warm, swollen, and tender, and the skin may turn purplish. Women are two to three times more likely to develop rheumatoid arthritis than are men. It can occur in young children, usually girls, but most often appears in people 40 years and older. Among elderly people it eventually may cause the joints to become misshapen as the ends of the bones enlarge and the muscles around them weaken.

Several causes of rheumatoid arthritis have been proposed, although no definitive cause has been identified. Many believe it is a type of autoimmune disorder, in which the body attacks itself—the connective tissue that supports the cartilage and joints—and causes the destruction of the joints. Some claim it is an immune reaction to a viral infection, a reaction to food allergies, or the result of faulty bowel permeability. According to Michael Murray, N.D., rheumatoid arthritis "is a classic example of a multi-factorial disease," in which various elements are responsible for the disease process.

Several other autoimmune diseases are similar to rheumatoid arthritis in that the connective tissue is affected. These include:

•*Ankylosing spondylitis* is inflammation of the synovial joints in the backbone and sometimes the hip and shoulder, resulting in pain and stiffness, and typically affecting people between the ages of 20 and 40.

•*Systemic lupus erythematosus* (also known as lupus) is characterized by extreme fatigue, severe muscle ache and joint pain, chest pain, rash, high sensitivity to the sun, blurred vision, swollen glands, nose and mouth ulcers, and low-grade fever. The first sign of the disease is usually a butterfly-shaped facial rash. Symptoms can affect any part of the body, and the course is unpredictable. Women are affected more often than men. Although the cause is unknown, factors such as sex hormones, heredity, and infection may be involved.

•*Polymyalgia rheumatica* is the presence of pain and stiffness in the muscles of the neck, arms, and shoulders or the back, thighs, and hips.

The natural treatment recommendations for these conditions are the same as those for rheumatoid arthritis.

Natural Remedies: Arnica, belladonna, boswellia, bromelain, bryonia, calcarea carbonica, cayenne (capsaicin), colocynthis, Chinese herbs, devil's claw, feverfew, ginger, magnesium, rhus toxicodendron, turmeric, white willow bark, magnet therapy, guided imagery.

Gout

Gout is signaled by the presence of sudden, intense pain in a joint, usually the big toe but also occurring in the ankle, knee, elbow, thumbs, or fingers. The pain usually, and unexplainably, happens in the middle of the night and may be accompanied by swelling, inflammation, and a feeling of heat in the affected joint. Gout is the accumulation of excess uric acid between the bones of these joints. Mild cases often can be controlled by diet, but chronic cases may require more aggressive treatment. Ninety percent of those afflicted with gout are men.

Natural Remedies: Arnica, bromelain, colocynthis, devil's claw, rhus toxicodendron.

Childhood Disorders

Several painful conditions that occur only or primarily in childhood can be treated very effectively with natural pain relievers. Dosing for children, especially infants, should be done only under a doctor's supervision. Because the belladonna plant is poisonous (though the homeopathic remedy is not), parents are warned to use only the homeopathic form of belladonna and to follow their health-care provider's instructions for use.

Colic

Colic is a painful gastrointestinal condition that typically first occurs in infants within the first six weeks of life and can last up to six months. Doctors diagnose colic if an otherwise healthy infant has the following behavior: persistent, loud crying that lasts three or more hours for three or more days a week over a three-week or longer period; drawing the legs up to the abdomen, curling the toes, and clenching the hands, all while crying; the infant's face alternately paling and flushing during the crying spells; prolonged crying between 6 P.M. and midnight from an infant that has been fed; and crying episodes that begin or end with flatulence or a bowel movement. Other symptoms include excessive spitting up of milk, burping, and gurgling noises.

Natural Remedies: Bryonia, colocynthis.

Ear Infections

Although not exclusive to childhood, ear infections and the accompanying earaches affect infants and children more often than they do adults: Approximately 95 percent of children get at least one ear infection by the time they reach age six. Otitis media, or middle ear infection, is the most common cause of earache. Symptoms include pain in the middle ear, high fever, nasal congestion, nausea and diarrhea, and pressure in the ear. If the infection is severe, it can lead to a ruptured eardrum. Otitis media usually is caused by inflammation of the Eustachian tube, the channel through which fluid and other substances drain out of the ear and into the throat. Inflammation typically occurs when the child gets a cold or flu. Environmental toxins, such as cigarette smoke, pollen, and fumes, also can cause inflammation. Yet another cause may be food allergies. More than 50 percent of children with chronic ear infections are allergic to specific foods, especially milk, wheat, and eggs.

Another common type of ear infection is otitis externa, or outer ear infection (swimmer's ear), in which the area from the eardrum to the outside of the ear becomes inflamed. Symptoms include fever, temporary loss of hearing in the affected ear, and a fluid discharge from the ear.

Natural Remedies: Belladonna, calcarea carbonica, St. John's wort.

Growing Pains

The sudden growth spurt that often occurs in adolescence, and more often in boys than in girls, is known as Osgood-Schlatter disease, or growing pains. The pain occurs below the kneecap and is accompanied by swelling. The condition is caused by the quadriceps muscle, which is in the front of the thigh, pulling on the tendon that attaches it to the shin. Often a tender lump can be felt below the kneecap. Growing pains typically last six months to a year. During that time, the affected child should refrain from jumping, running, and squatting.

Natural Remedy: Calcarea phosphorica.

Teething

A child's 20 baby teeth usually begin to emerge gradually starting at age four months, when the teeth move toward the gum surface. At around seven months the first teeth appear, and the entire process is usually over by age 24 to 30 months. Although teething is a natural development, it can be painful for the child and distressing for the parents. Symptoms of teething include an increase in fussing and crying at night, drooling and chewing on fingers, swollen gums, and refusal to breast- or bottle-feed.

Natural Remedies: Belladonna, calcarea carbonica.

Gynecologic Conditions

~~~~~

Dysmenorrhea (Painful Menstruation)

Painful periods are a very common condition among women, but that doesn't make it any less painful and occasionally debilitating for one or more days per month. Painful periods usually are caused by an excess of prostaglandins, hormonelike substances that can cause the uterus to contract and result in menstrual cramping. Dysmenorrhea also may be caused by endometriosis, the abnormal growth of uterine tissue on the outside of the uterus and often on the ovaries, fallopian tubes, and other surrounding tissue. This abnormal tissue bleeds, and because the blood cannot escape as menstrual blood does normally during a woman's cycle, it forms adhesions, which eventually form scar tissue and results in chronic pain. Endometriosis affects approximately 5 million American girls and women between the ages of 11 and 50 and is the number-one reason for infertility and hysterectomy.

Natural Remedies: Belladonna, bromelain, calcarea phosphorica, colocynthis, Chinese herbs, devil's claw, St. John's wort, magnesium, marijuana, turmeric, white willow bark; biofeedback, magnet therapy, meditation.

Pelvic Inflammatory Disease

The term "pelvic inflammatory disease" (PID) is used to describe a bacterial infection that affects any of the organs in a woman's pelvic region, including the uterus, fallopian tubes, and ovaries. PID can be either acute or chronic. Symptoms of an acute PID include sudden onset of severe pain and tenderness in the lower abdomen, vaginal discharge, and occasionally fever. Chronic cases involve a low-grade infection that causes mild but recurring pain, backache, pain during intercourse, a heavy vaginal discharge, and irregular menstrual cycle. Symptoms may be so mild that a woman may not realize she has the disease until she tries to become pregnant and discovers she is infertile, which is a common result of a PID that is not treated.

Natural Remedy: Belladonna.

Premenstrual Syndrome (PMS)

Premenstrual syndrome is a condition characterized by various physical and emotional symptoms that typically occur a week to 10 days before the menstrual period begins. PMS is believed to affect up to 50 percent of women regularly, and up to 10 percent of women have symptoms severe enough to cause them to seek medical help. More than 150 symptoms have been identified with PMS, some of which include breast swelling and pain, headache, backache, joint and muscle pain, bloating and fluid retention, acne, weight gain, moodiness, anxiety, food cravings, insomnia, drowsiness, hot flashes, constipation, and diarrhea.

The exact cause of PMS is unknown, although many theories have been proposed to explain the symptoms associated with the condition. Some believe a hormone imbalance is to blame; others cite dietary deficiencies (vitamin B_6, essential fatty acids, magnesium), fluctuations of certain brain chemicals, and genetics.

Natural Remedies: Boswellia, calcarea carbonica, Chinese herbs, magnesium; meditation.

Childbirth

Childbirth here refers to labor pains as well as episiotomy (an incision made to enlarge the vaginal opening) and cesarean section. Several natural approaches can be used, with your doctor's knowledge, to ease the pain of giving birth and aid in postpartum recovery.

Natural Remedies: Arnica, Chinese herbs; self-hypnosis.

Fibromyalgia

Fibromyalgia is in a classification by itself because the pain is so widespread and affects so many different bodily systems that it does not fit into any one of the other categories. According to the American College of Rheumatology, the criteria for fibromyalgia are a history of widespread pain for at least three months; six or more typical, reproducible tender points; and exclusion of other diseases or conditions that cause the same symptoms. Many people who have fibromyalgia also fulfill some or all of the following criteria: chronic headache, painful menstruation, irritable bowel, generalized fatigue, disturbed sleep, swollen joints, tingling or numbing sensations in the arms and legs, and urinary tract infections.

The primary cause of the exaggerated pain associated with fibromyalgia is a chronically low level of serotonin, a hormone produced in the brain that regulates nerve impulses. Thus one of the best ways to control the pain of fibromyalgia is to increase serotonin levels, and the natural remedy that may do this best is **5-HTP**.

Natural Remedies: Arnica, boswellia, bryonia, 5-HTP, magnesium, MSM, St. John's wort; magnet therapy, meditation, guided imagery.

Headache and Migraine

Along with back pain, headaches are one of the most common pains suffered by Americans. More than 45 million suffer with headache every year, and they spend more than $4 billion trying to make headaches go away. The majority of headaches are a result of tension, which causes the blood vessels in the head to constrict. The pain is typically persistent and dull and affects both sides of the head. Tension headache is precipitated by physical or emotional stress, anxiety, eye strain, dehydration, PMS, lack of sleep, or food allergy. It is sometimes related to consumption of caffeine, alcohol, or drugs.

One common cause of tension headache that is often overlooked is the routine use of over-the-counter analgesics. For some tension headache sufferers, the habitual use of these drugs results in their being less effective and leads to a syndrome called rebound headache, in which the very drugs designed to eliminate the pain actually perpetuate it. If you are taking OTC drugs daily for chronic head pain and getting little or no relief, you likely have rebound headache. Use of natural pain relievers, while gradually withdrawing from conventional drugs with the aid of your physician, may be the answer to your headache problems.

Approximately 17 percent of American women and 6 percent of men suffer with migraine headache, a severe, recurring (one to four times a month on average) pain that usually affects one side of the head. Nausea, vomiting, lightheadedness, tingling or numbness in the arms or head, and visual disturbances called auras often accompany attacks of migraine pain. The pain is often debilitating and can last 4 to 72 hours.

A less common type of headache pain, but one that is severe, is **cluster headache**. Men are 10 times more likely to experience this type of pain, which usually occurs on one side of the head and recurs in clusters over weeks or months. The pain typically lasts about one hour and usually is accompanied by runny nose, watery eyes, and swelling below the eye on the affected side.

Natural Remedies:

For migraine: Chinese herbs, feverfew, 5-HTP, ginger, magnesium, marijuana, St. John's wort; biofeedback, self-hypnosis.

For tension headache: Arnica, belladonna, bromelain, bryonia, calcarea carbonica, calcarea phosphorica, colocynthis, Chinese herbs, devil's claw, 5-HTP, ginger, MSM, rhus toxicodendron, white willow bark; biofeedback, magnet therapy, meditation, self-hypnosis.

For cluster headache: Cayenne (capsaicin), magnesium.

Muscle, Trauma, and Related-to-Overuse Pain

Pain associated with muscle weakness or injury (e.g., backache), trauma associated with sports injuries or accidents (e.g., abrasions, bruises, sprains, strains, fractures, dislocations), and overuse, such as bursitis, tendonitis, fibrositis, and carpal tunnel syndrome, are included in this category.

Backache
The most common physical complaint among American adults is back pain. At any one time, 16 percent of people between the ages of 25 and 74 years have lower back pain. Approximately 2 percent of the entire U.S. population is either temporarily or permanently disabled with back pain.

The primary cause of back pain is weak muscles in the back and abdomen. Because the muscles are in a weakened state, overexertion, improper lifting, prolonged sitting, and bad posture are often the factors that trigger the pain. Prevention of back pain includes exercises to strengthen back and abdominal muscles and maintaining good posture and lifting habits.

A condition known as fibrositis is one of the most common causes of back pain. Fibrositis is characterized by small adhesions that lie between individual muscle fibers. These adhesions typically are caused by repetitive or habitual strain associated with poor posture and work habits and emotional tension as well as weak back and abdominal muscles. When muscles are in a weakened state, overexertion, improper lifting, prolonged sitting or standing in one spot, and bad posture can trigger back pain. Prevention of back pain can be achieved with exercises to strengthen back and abdominal muscles and by maintaining good posture and lifting habits.

Natural Remedies: Arnica, boswellia, bromelain, bryonia, calcarea carbonica, calcarea phosphorica, Chinese herbs, devil's claw, hypericum, MSM, rhus toxicodendron, white willow bark; biofeedback, magnet therapy, meditation.

Bursitis

Bursitis is an inflammation of the bursa, a saclike membrane that contains a fluid which lubricates the joints. The inflammation, pain, and swelling occurs most often in the elbow, lower knee, shoulder, and hip. Injury, infection, strain, and arthritis are the usual causes of bursitis. Athletes who engage in running, throwing, jumping, or any type of repetitive motion can get bursitis, as can people with jobs that require strenuous or repetitive activity. Bursitis usually resolves in a few days or weeks if the affected area is rested. Repeat attacks of bursitis can lead to chronic cases in which calcium deposits in the tissues can permanently reduce mobility.

Natural Remedies: Belladonna, bryonia, glucosamine, MSM, rhus toxicodendron, white willow bark; magnet therapy.

Carpal Tunnel Syndrome

Carpal tunnel syndrome is an overuse disorder (sometimes called a repetitive stress injury) characterized by shooting pains in the forearm, wrist, and occasionally to the shoulder, neck, and chest; numbness or tingling in the hand; difficulty grasping small objects or clenching the fist; and, in some cases, dry skin and deterioration of the fingernails. It is usually the result of repetitive manual activity, such as keyboarding, operating power tools, playing some musical instruments, and hammering. Sports that may cause carpal tunnel syndrome include rowing, golf, tennis, and rock climbing.

Natural Remedies: Boswellia, bromelain, MSM, rhus toxicodendron; magnet therapy.

Muscle Pain

Included in this category are painful conditions that involve the muscles and that often are related to sports injuries, such as strains, sprains, bruises, and cramps.

Natural Remedies: Arnica, bromelain, calcarea carbonica, cayenne (capsaicin), Chinese herbs, ginger, magnesium, marijuana, MSM, rhus toxicodendron; magnet therapy.

Tendonitis

Tendonitis is an inflammation of a tendon, the connective tissue that connects muscles to bones. Strain is the usual cause, and the resulting pain can be acute or chronic and cause the affected area to have a limited range of motion. The tendons most often affected are the biceps, the back of the ankle, the knee, the inside of the foot, and the rotator cuff in the shoulder. Acute cases usually heal within a few days to a few weeks; chronic cases can be more difficult if individuals continue to strain the affected tendons.

Natural Remedies: Belladonna, glucosamine, MSM, rhus toxicodendron; magnet therapy.

Trauma

Types of trauma include fractures, dislocations, abrasions, and torn ligaments. These painful conditions often are the result of an accident, such as falls or automobile mishaps.

Natural Remedies: Arnica, bromelain, calcarea carbonica, calcarea phosphorica, hypericum (homeopathic remedy), St. John's wort (herb).

Neurological Pain

The painful conditions listed below involve inflammation, irritation, or malfunction of the nerves.

Neuralgia

Neuralgia, or nerve pain, is an umbrella term for several types of pain that occur when a nerve is inflamed or irritated. The pain may be sudden, sharp, stabbing, burning, or shooting, and it may last several seconds or a few minutes. Some people have occasional attacks; others suffer with chronic pain. There are three common types of neuralgia: trigeminal neuralgia, sciatica, and shingles. Diabetic neuropathy is another common nerve disorder that is associated with a great deal of pain.

•*Trigeminal neuralgia,* also known as *tic doloreux*, is a malfunction of the trigeminal nerve, which is located along the side of the face. It carries nerve impulses from the face to the brain. The pain associated with trigeminal neuralgia occurs in the lower portion of the face, usually in the cheek next to the nose. It is brief but excruciating, lasting several seconds to several minutes and recurring up to 100 times a day. The cause is unknown, and there is no cure. People of all ages can get this disorder, but it is most common among people older than 50, and it affects women three times more often than men.

Natural Remedies: Cayenne (capsaicin), colocynthis.

•*Sciatica* is a pain that radiates from the lower back (the lumbosacral area) down one or both buttocks, hips, or legs along the sciatic nerve. The pain can be shooting, sharp, or dull, and intermittent or continuous. Some people also experience numbness and weakness on the affected side. Sciatica occurs when the sciatic nerve at the base of the spine is compressed because of poor posture, pregnancy, a slipped disk, muscle strain, obesity, wearing high heels, or sleeping on a too-soft mattress. Seek medical attention if the pain lasts for more than three or four days and you are also experiencing leg or foot weakness.

Natural Remedies: Boswellia, colocynthis, Chinese herbs, rhus toxicodendron, white willow bark.

•*Shingles* and *Postherpetic neuralgia* are considered together because one (postherpetic neuralgia) generally follows the other (shingles). Shingles is the reactivation of the herpes zoster virus, the same virus that causes chicken pox, in adults. After children experience chicken pox, the virus lies dormant in the spinal nerve cells, where it can be stimulated into action years later when the immune system becomes compromised. Scientists do not know why this virus resurfaces in some people and not others. The first symptoms of shingles are a slight fever, and a tingling sensation or pain on one side of the body, followed in a few days by a rash and clusters of blisters. The affected areas are often very painful and itchy. The blisters usually heal in about two weeks and form scabs, but the pain continues. Postherpetic neuralgia is pain that continues beyond one month even if the rash is gone. The pain is typically deep, searing, aching, or stabbing. No treatment has been found either to prevent or to stop shingles or postherpetic neuralgia.

Natural Remedies: Cayenne (capsaicin), rhus toxicodendron.

Diabetic Neuropathy

Diabetic neuropathy, a common complication of diabetes, involves the loss of nerve function in peripheral areas of the body, especially the feet. Occasionally it also affects internal organs such as the heart and bladder. Nerve damage from diabetic neuropathy can cause pain, numbness, tingling sensations, or weakness in the muscles. Cuts, blisters, bruises, and other injuries may occur and go unnoticed because the person cannot feel the pain, which sometimes can lead to serious infection.

Natural Remedy: Cayenne (capsaicin).

Postsurgical Pain

Surgery, whether elective (as in cosmetic procedures) or necessary, places significant stress on the body by traumatizing the circulatory and nervous systems and compromising the immune system. Postsurgical patients are routinely given narcotic painkillers, which drug the nerves and typically cause troublesome side effects. The use of natural pain relievers both before and after surgery can significantly reduce or in some cases eliminate the need for conventional painkillers.

Natural Remedies: Arnica, bromelain, cayenne (capsaicin), hypericum; guided imagery, meditation.

Other Painful Conditions

Burns
Exposure to heat greater than 120° Fahrenheit causes damage to skin cells, resulting in burns graded from

first to fourth degree. A first-degree burn results in red, tender skin with possible swelling and minor blistering. Sunburn often falls into this classification. A second-degree burn is more serious and is painful. The skin is very red and blistered. If the skin is white or charred and you can see blood vessels, or the nerves are exposed and there is no pain, the burn is third degree. If bone and muscle are exposed, the burn is fourth degree. The natural remedies discussed in this book are for first- and most second-degree burns only; all others should be treated immediately by a physician. Second-degree burns that affect a large portion of the body or that develop an infection also should be treated by a physician.

Natural Remedies: St. John's wort, white willow bark; self-hypnosis.

Cystitis

Cystitis (or urinary tract infection) is an inflammation of the bladder that is accompanied by a burning sensation or pain when urinating, a frequent urge to urinate, and urine with a strong odor. It is very common in women and rare in men. The most common cause of cystitis is infection by strains of *Escherichia coli*, bacteria normally found in the intestines. Scientists speculate that because women have a shorter urethra (the tube that transports urine from the bladder) and the vaginal and anal openings are close to the urethra, it is easy for bacteria to be transported to the bladder.

A chronic, nonbacterial form of the disease is interstitial cystitis, which is characterized by pain in the pelvic area, back pain, painful sexual intercourse, and urinary frequency. The cause is unknown.

Natural Remedies: Belladonna, MSM.

Gallbladder Disorders

The gallbladder, a pear-shape organ that stores the digestive juices (bile), is prone to the development of deposits called gallstones. Ten percent of the people in the United States will have one or more gallstones at some point in their lives. Gallstones can be as small as a grain of sand or as big as a golfball. Most people with gallstones don't have symptoms. Gallstones can float in the gallbladder for as long as 25 years before they become a problem. Symptoms of severe and sudden pain in the upper right abdomen and into the back, severe nausea and vomiting, indigestion, and fever are an indication that the stones have become lodged in the cystic duct, a small canal that joins the gallbladder to the common bile duct. An obstructed duct can cause inflammation, infection, and eventually liver damage if left untreated for years.

Natural Remedy: Devil's claw.

Hemorrhoids

Hemorrhoids are a form of varicose veins that affect the rectum and anus. Symptoms of hemorrhoids include pain, presence of bright red blood that streaks the feces or toilet tissue, pain during bowel movements, anal itching, painful swelling near the anus, and a mucus discharge from the anus. Hemorrhoids can be either internal or external. Internal hemorrhoids usually do not hurt because there are few pain-receptor nerves in the rectum. If they become enlarged (prolapse), they may protrude from the anus and become painful. External hemorrhoids are usually painful because the anus has many pain-sensing nerves.

Natural Remedies: Belladonna, Chinese herbs, St. John's wort.

Irritable Bowel Syndrome

Irritable bowel syndrome is a very common digestive condition that affects 10 to 15 percent of adults at some time during their lives. The symptoms reported most often are abdominal pain and diarrhea; other people experience painful constipation and abdominal cramps, usually after eating. Symptoms may last for several weeks. The cause of irritable bowel syndrome is not known, although it appears to be stress related. Other factors that seem to cause or aggravate symptoms include overeating, a high-fat diet, smoking, and lactose intolerance.

Natural Remedies: St. John's wort, turmeric; meditation.

Sinusitis

Sinusitis is an infection or inflammation of the sinuses, the four pairs of hollow chambers in the bones of the face. This condition affects up to 50 million Americans a year. Mucus forms on the surface of the sinuses, which traps dirt and other particles that are inhaled. The particles are then pushed through openings in the sinuses called ostia. When these openings become inflamed or clogged, the sinuses swell and become infected.

Symptoms of sinusitis include pressure and a feeling of pain and fullness behind the eyes, difficulty breathing through the nose, and postnasal drip. Some people also experience fever and a toothache. The most common triggers of sinusitis are upper respiratory tract viral infections, allergic reactions, and hay fever. If your sinus infection does not improve in seven days, or if you get three or more attacks of sinusitis a year and they occur closer and closer together, call your doctor, as chronic sinusitis can lead to more serious problems, such as bronchitis or pneumonia.

Natural Remedies: Bromelain, Chinese herbs.

Temporomandibular Joint Syndrome

Up to two-thirds of Americans will have some symptoms of temporomandibular joint syndrome, or TMJ, during their lifetime. TMJ, also known as myofascial pain dysfunction, is a condition in which the temporomandibular joint, which joins the jawbone to the skull, causes pain in front of the ears and in the facial muscles. The most common cause of TMJ is excessive stress on the jaw muscles, caused by grinding the teeth during sleep, head injury, an uncorrected bite, poorly fitting dentures, or arthritis. People with TMJ often feel a popping sensation when they open their mouth or may feel pain when they open their mouth. Some also have recurring headache.

Natural Remedies: Biofeedback, self-hypnosis, meditation, guided imagery, magnet therapy.

Thrombophlebitis

Thrombophlebitis is a condition that involves inflammation of the veins and the formation of blood clots (or thrombi). These clots cause pain and may block the flow of blood in the affected veins.

There are two types of thrombophlebitis: superficial and deep. The superficial form is the more common type and is characterized by a red, swollen vein in the leg that is hard, tender, and warm. The skin may feel as if it is throbbing or burning, and there is pain and heaviness when the leg is lowered. Deep thrombophlebitis is less common but more dangerous. The deep interior veins are affected, and because they are bigger than the veins that are closer to the skin surface, they have the potential to carry larger blood clots. These clots can be transported to the lungs, where they may prove fatal.

Possible causes of or contributing factors for thrombophlebitis include already having varicose veins, infection, trauma, gender (approximately 70 percent of people with thrombophlebitis are women), use of oral contraceptives, obesity, sedentary lifestyle, and smoking.

Natural Remedy: Bromelain.

Toothache

Tooth pain can be caused by: an acute or chronic infection of the gums or the underlying support structures of the teeth; tooth decay that has caused a cavity to form; or teeth that have grown at an angle (impacted teeth). Typical symptoms are a sharp or aching pain in the affected tooth when you chew or bite, often accompanied by sore gums or an aching jaw. Other signs of tooth decay are a tooth that is extremely sensitive to heat or cold or one that feels as if it is throbbing. Tooth decay that is not remedied quickly may develop into an abscess, an infection below the gum that requires emergency treatment.

Natural Remedies: Arnica, belladonna, bryonia, calcarea carbonica, Chinese herbs, rhus toxicodendron; self-hypnosis.

Ulcers

An ulcer is a painful, craterlike erosion of the stomach lining or the duodenum (part of the small intestine) usually caused by the bacteria *Helicobactor pylori*. The pain can be aching or gnawing and occurs just before or several hours after eating. Sometimes the pain is accompanied by nausea, vomiting, indigestion, or weight loss. If you notice blood in your stools or in your vomit, call your physician immediately.

Natural Remedies: Boswellia; meditation.

Now that you are armed with a better understanding of different painful conditions and the names of natural pain relievers for each of them, it's time to learn about those painkillers. Chapters 4 and 5 provide the information you need to control your pain naturally, safely, and effectively.

	Back pain	Burns	Bursitis and tendonitis	Cancer pain	Carpal tunnel syndrome	Childbirth	Cluster headache	Colic	Cystitis	Diabetic neuropathy	Dysmenorrhea	Ear infection	Fibromyalgia	Glaucoma	Gallbladder disorders
ARNICA	•					•							•		
BELLADONNA			•						•		•	•			
BOSWELLIA	•				•								•		
BROMELAIN	•				•						•				
BRYONIA	•							•					•		
CALCAREA CARBONICA	•											•			
CALCAREA PHOSPHORICA	•										•				
CAYENNE (CAPSAICIN)							•			•					
COLOCYNTHIS								•							
CHINESE HERBS	•					•					•				
DEVIL'S CLAW	•										•				•
FEVERFEW															
5-HTP													•		
GINGER															
GLUCOSAMINE			•												
HYPERICUM	•										•		•		
MAGNESIUM								•			•		•		
MARIJUANA											•			•	
MSM	•		•	•					•				•		
RHUS TOXICODENDRON	•		•	•											
ST. JOHN'S WORT		•									•	•	•		
TURMERIC				•							•				
WHITE WILLOW BARK	•	•									•				
BIOFEEDBACK	•			•							•				
HYPNOSIS		•		•		•									
MAGNET THERAPY	•		•	•	•						•		•		
MEDITATION	•			•							•		•		
VISUALIZATION/ GUIDED IMAGERY				•									•		

Gout	Growing pains	Headache	Hemorrhoids	Irritable bowel syndrome	Liver disorders	Migraine	Muscle pain	Neuralgia	Osteoarthritis	Pelvic inflammatory disease	Postsurgical pain	Premenstrual syndrome	Rheumatoid arthritis	Sciatica	Shingles	Sinusitis	Teething	Thrombophlebitis	TMJ	Trauma pain	Trigeminal neuralgia	Toothache	Ulcers
●		●					●		●		●												
		●	●						●	●			●				●					●	
									●			●	●	●									●
●		●					●		●		●		●			●		●		●			
		●																				●	
		●					●	●				●	●			●				●			
	●	●					●																
							●	●				●			●						●		
●		●	●				●	●				●	●			●						●	
●		●			●		●	●	●														
							●																
							●																
									●														
			●				●				●									●			
							●	●				●											
							●	●	●														
		●					●	●	●														
●		●					●	●	●				●	●	●							●	
				●			●						●							●			
			●	●	●								●										
		●						●	●						●								
		●				●													●				
		●				●													●				
		●					●	●					●						●			●	
		●	●									●	●						●				●
							●	●					●							●			

CHAPTER FOUR

Nature's Most Powerful Pain Relievers

Pain is older than humankind, and so are ways to relieve it. Long before we depended on the synthetic chemical concoctions that crowd our drugstore shelves and monopolize the lives of many individuals who live with chronic pain today, people sought relief from Nature's bounty. Instead of picking up a prescription from the corner pharmacy, they picked local herbs. Rather than pop pill after pill full of substances few people can even pronounce, they drank teas and chewed the leaves of plants that were their friends.

This chapter and the next introduce you to some of those friends—some you may have heard of before, others may be new to you. This chapter contains detailed information about natural pain relievers from the worlds of herbal medicine (Western and Chinese) and homeopathy, as well as several natural supplements. The remedies discussed are among those most effective in the relief of pain, especially chronic pain. All of them have undergone at least some scientific scrutiny, and relevant findings have been included with each entry. In many cases, anecdotal reports overwhelmingly support the use of the remedy for pain relief. Arguably, other natural substances could be added to this list. Indeed, sometimes another herb, supplement, or homeopathic remedy is mentioned as an adjunct to the ones explained here at length. You are invited to explore them by referring to the Bibliography and Suggested Reading list.

The "How to Use It" section in each entry contains dosing instructions for specific diseases and conditions as well as general recommendations where applicable. The general information can help you better understand the remedies and how to get the most benefit from them. If any of the terms used in the entries are unfamiliar to you, turn to the Glossary at the end of the book. Once you have chosen the natural pain reliever that best fits your needs, turn to Chapter 6 for help in buying and using your remedy.

Herbal Remedies

Herbal medicine is a system of natural healing that uses plants and their extracts to treat physical and mental conditions. It has been practiced in every culture since recorded history, and probably even earlier. An important principle of herbal medicine is "synergism," which means that the strength of the sum of an herb's parts is greater than the effectiveness of any of its individual components. Thus even though many conventional drugs contain one or several active ingredients derived from herbs, herbalists explain that the power of herbal remedies is attributable to the fact that Nature intended for *all* of an herb's dozens or even hundreds of components to work together, with each having a definite role in the healing process and in preventing adverse effects.

Herbal remedies are available in many forms. The ones discussed in this book include tablets, capsules, infusions, decoctions, extracts, and tinctures. Any one of these forms can be *standardized*, a term that means the herb is guaranteed to contain a standard amount of certain active components. Standardization is practiced widely in Europe and less so in the United States, although more and more U.S. herbal products are being standardized. When purchasing herbs, look for standardized formulas: They are the forms most likely to provide you with the amount of active ingredients you need.

Tablets and *capsules* are composed of powdered or finely milled herbal material. Some tablets are enteric-coated, which means that a special protein-based coating has been applied that allows the tablet to retain its components until it reaches the small intestine, where it can be absorbed without being damaged by acids in the stomach. If swallowing capsules is a problem, in many cases they can be broken open and the contents added to liquid or food.

Infusions are prepared like teas, but they use more of the herb than do other teas and they are allowed to steep longer to achieve greater potency. Infusions are made from the leaves, flowers, and other soft parts of the plant. They can be taken hot or cold, depending on the herb and its indicated use.

Decoctions are similar to infusions except they use the hard part of the plant—roots, stems, and bark. Because these plant parts are tougher, they need to steep longer than do infusions.

Extracts are made from the juice of the crushed plant, mixed with a small amount of water. They are more potent than infusions and decoctions and have a higher concentration of active ingredients.

Tinctures are extracts that are mixed with alcohol instead of water. They usually are made from herbs that, for some reason, are not suitable for infusions or decoctions, such as arnica.

Homeopathic Remedies

Homeopathy is a system of medicine in which remedies are taken to stimulate and promote the body's own natural healing abilities. The remedies it uses are capable of producing symptoms in a healthy person similar to those present in a patient who needs the remedy. If a healthy person were given the homeopathic remedy bryonia, for example, she would experience vertigo, eyes that burned and felt like they were full of dust; tearing pain in the neck, back, and limbs; frontal headache; and early-morning diarrhea. If a person went to a homeopath complaining of these symptoms, he/she would likely prescribe bryonia.

Homeopathy is also a system in which less is more:

The less actual substance present in a remedy, the more powerful the remedy is purported to be. This concept places homeopathy in the category of an energy therapy, which means the remedies work at the energy level, not at the level of matter. (For further details about homeopathy, see the Bibliography and Suggested Reading list.)

How to Pick a Homeopathic Remedy

Homeopathic remedies are chosen by matching a person's individual characteristics and symptoms with the characteristics of a particular remedy. For example, belladonna can relieve menstrual cramps that resemble labor pains and those that improve when bending over or lying down. Women who benefit best from belladonna are sturdy and typically of robust health. If you are experiencing menstrual cramps but are lean and feel relief when you are warm, colocynthis may be better for you, as these characteristics match this remedy. The more individual symptoms and characteristics you can match with a particular remedy, the more likely it is to give you relief. To help you match your qualities with those of the different homeopathic remedies, all the homeopathic entries in the section that follows have a separate heading called "Matching Characteristics."

In the United States, homeopathic remedies are generally prepared according to the "centesimal" (hundred) or "c" scale. In the "How to Use It" sections for homeopathic remedies, you will see instructions to take "30c" or "6c" of a remedy. The "c" indicates how much the remedy was diluted. A 1c remedy consists of 1 part substance and 99 parts water (or water and alcohol). A 30c dose is more potent than a 6c dose. For guidelines on how to take homeopathic remedies, including the Rule of Three, see page 220.

How Do Homeopathic Remedies Work?

An explanation as to how oral homeopathic remedies are effective apparently lies with the three general principles set forth by the founder of homeopathy, Samuel Hahnemann. One principle is the Law of Similars, which says that a substance that can cause symptoms of illness in a healthy person can eliminate those same or similar symptoms in a person who is ill when that substance is taken in minuscule amounts. The second principle, Minimum Dose, states that repeated dilution of the substance increases rather than decreases its potency while it eliminates the risk of adverse effects. The third principle says that remedies must be prescribed for the specific needs of each individual, based on a person's physical and emotional state, personality, diet, lifestyle, temperament, and other distinguishing characteristics.

Proving That Homeopathy Works

Many conventional medicine professionals are skeptical about the effectiveness of homeopathic remedies. This skepticism stems from a lack of understanding about homeopathy and a firm belief that one must put a substance through rigorously controlled trials and scientifically measure the evidence before declaring it "effective." Homeopaths themselves do not understand how homeopathic remedies work, yet for the past 200 years they have seen evidence of it every day in the patients they treat. And because people in glass houses should be the last one to throw stones, contemporary physicians and pharmacologists admit that they are uncertain about exactly why many of the most commonly used drugs on the market today, including antibiotics and aspirin, work. Yet this lack of knowledge does not prevent them from freely prescribing and recommending them. When you combine these facts with the high incidence of adverse side effects often caused by conventional medications and the lack of such effects associated with homeopathic remedies, you may begin to have a healthy skepticism yourself about many conventional medications.

One concept of conventional medicine is "more is better"—the larger the dose, the more powerful the effect will be. Yet knowledgeable medical professionals know this is not true. According to a pharmacological principle known as the Arndt-Schultz law (named after the two researchers who discovered it in the 1870s), rather than a drug producing greater effects as the dose is increased, exceedingly small doses actually have greater effects than large doses. In other words, the two researchers found that while high concentrations of a substance inhibit healing, low concentrations stimulate it. This phenomenon was named "homnesis" in the 1920s and has since been verified by hundreds of studies conducted by conventional scientists. Yet although homnesis is consistent with homeopathic principles, scientists have largely refused to apply this concept to test the extremely high dilutions used in homeopathy.

Another obstacle to homeopathic research is that, like herbs, homeopathic remedies are natural substances and cannot be patented. Pharmaceutical companies, which finance and ultimately profit from marketing their drugs, are not interested in spending time and money on testing substances for which they cannot make money.

A difficulty with scientifically testing homeopathic remedies is that homeopathy is inherently individualistic: A remedy is prescribed based on numerous personal traits. Ten people who have a cold may be prescribed 10 different homeopathic remedies based on their personality, lifestyle, and other factors. In conventional medicine, those 10 people would all receive the same remedy. Thus it is virtually impossible to conduct a controlled study of homeopathic remedies of any significant size unless you found a group of people who were exactly alike.

All of this introduces the fact that there is little clinical research on the effectiveness of homeopathy in the area of pain management. Each of the entries in this chapter have a heading called "Here's the Proof." For homeopathic entries, any published scientific studies on the particular remedy will be explained under this heading. However, despite the lack of published reports, there have been and continue to be countless anecdotal reports of the efficacy of these homeopathic remedies.

In 1991 a group of scientists (none of them homeopaths) from the Netherlands reviewed all controlled trials of homeopathic medicine done over a 25-year period. According to their results, published in the *British Medical Journal*, of the 107 controlled trials evaluated, 81 showed that homeopathic remedies were effective, 24 indicated they were ineffective, and 2 drew no definite conclusions. Of the studies relating to pain, 18 of 20 showed improvement in the treatment of pain or trauma, 4 of 6 showed benefit in the treatment of arthritis and rheumatoid disorders, and 13 of 15 showed improvement in miscellaneous disorders, including headache and neurological conditions. Overall, the researchers concluded that "[t]he evidence . . . would probably be sufficient for establishing homeopathy as a regular treatment for certain indications."

How Safe Are Homeopathic Remedies?

Homeopathic remedies are very safe when taken in low potencies. (Up to 30c is considered low potency.) In homeopathy, the quality and frequency of dosing is what matters, and not the quantity of remedy taken. Many people self-treat with homeopathic remedies for the conditions discussed in the individual entries for remedies that follow.

Nature's Painkillers

The following is an alphabetical list of herbs, homeopathic remedies, and supplements used to treat pain. Speak with your physician before you start any pain relief program. Always consult your pediatrician before administering any remedy to children.

Arnica

What Is Arnica?
Arnica is a perennial herb of the family *Compositae*. It grows about one foot tall and is found in the higher elevations of Europe and northern Asia and in some parts of the northwestern United States. It is also known as mountain daisy, mountain arnica, wolfsbane, and leopard's bane. Its pain relief qualities have long been appreciated by mountain climbers in the Alps, who chew arnica to relieve muscle aches and pain after long hikes. In early nineteenth-century Europe, arnica was used topically to treat cuts, sprains, and bruises. The entire plant, including its yellow flowers, is used to make the homeopathic remedy, which is available as a tincture and a topical cream.

What Types of Pain Does Arnica Help?
- Childbirth
- Fibromyalgia

- Gout
- Headache
- Muscle pain
- Osteoarthritis
- Postsurgical
- Rheumatoid arthritis
- Toothache
- Trauma

Matching Characteristics

People who benefit most from arnica are generally morose and morbidly imaginative. They usually refuse medical care regardless of how sick they are, and they prefer to be left alone. Restlessness, feelings of hopelessness, impatience, sleeplessness, and absent-mindedness are typical characteristics. They also may be prone to nightmares and a horror of instant death. Accompanying symptoms that indicate arnica use include dry mouth, feeble pulse, swollen joints, and pain in the limbs and back. People may experience a hot head and a cold body and have great thirst during their chill. Heat, rest, and light pressure on the affected sites usually make symptoms worse; symptoms improve when people first begin to move around but worsen as they continue to move.

How Do You Use Arnica?

Arnica should be taken as soon as possible after experiencing an injury. Arnica remedies are available in tincture, granule, lotion, ointment, powder, and tablet form. Look for arnica ointment with a maximum concentration of 15 percent arnica oil. Tablets and lotion are the most common forms, but any one is equally effective when taken according to the Rule of Three. (See page 200.) If taking a tablet, place it under the tongue and allow it to dissolve. See Chapter 6 for dosing instructions for children. Alternative dosages for several specific conditions follow.

•**Back Pain (Lower):** Use arnica when there is severe back pain after an injury. The affected area can feel bruised and may be swollen. Take 30c every hour for up to 10 doses. An alternative approach is to take 6c four times daily for up to two days, and apply a topical arnica gel or ointment.

•**Bruises:** Take 30c two to three times daily for several days. Arnica works best if taken before the skin begins to turn black and blue.

•**Childbirth:** Take 30c right before delivery to reduce pain and speed up recovery. Consult with your obstetrician before using arnica for this purpose.

•**Fibromyalgia:** Arnica is indicated when the muscles feel as if you slept on a too-hard bed and the pain is worse when you move. Take 30c every three hours for up to two days.

•**Fractures:** Take one to two 200c-doses immediately after injury, then take 30c two to three times daily for several days.

•**Gout:** Arnica is indicated when joints are painful and feel bruised. Take 30c every 15 minutes, up to 10 doses.

•**Headache:** For cases in which the head feels

bruised and aching and the pain is worse when stooping. There may be occasional sharp pain. Take 30c every 10 to 15 minutes for up to 10 doses.

•**Muscle Pain:** Treat with arnica immediately after the injury. Apply ointment to the affected area. (Caution: Do not apply to broken skin.) This can be in addition to oral dosing. If the muscles have been pulled or strained, take 30c immediately after the injury every hour for up to six doses. Thereafter, take 30c four times daily for up to three days. If you get little or no relief, take **rhus toxicodendron.** (See page 150.)

•**Osteoarthritis:** Arnica is helpful for flare-ups but not for chronic pain and in cases where joint pain is the consequence of or made worse by an injury. Take 30c four times daily for up to two weeks, and apply the ointment as needed.

•**Postsurgery (Including Dental Surgery):** Take 30c before and 200c immediately upon awakening after the procedure to reduce pain and promote healing. Repeat the 200c dose two to three times until the pain subsides. If shooting pain associated with nerve damage occurs, follow the arnica treatment with **hypericum.** (See page 131.)

How Does Arnica Work?

In the early 1980s, investigators in Germany identified two substances in arnica—helanalin and dihydrohelanalin—responsible for reducing inflammation and pain. These substances appear to be present at sufficient levels in the ointment to be effective against pain. Some reports claim that arnica ointment can stimulate reabsorption of blood and significantly reduce bruising and also counteract shock and emotional trauma that may be related to the injury. For additional details, see page 61.

Here's the Proof
See the explanation on page 61.

How Safe Is Arnica?
See the explanation on page 64.

Belladonna

What Is Belladonna?
Atropa belladonna, also known as deadly nightshade, is a plant with yellow flowers and dark red berries that grows wild in Europe. Belladonna, which means "beautiful woman" in Italian, gets its name from the Renaissance era when Italian ladies placed belladonna drops in their eyes to achieve a doe-eyed appearance and rubbed it on their skin to remove pimples.

Before Samuel Hahnemann added belladonna to his arsenal of homeopathic remedies, it was used medicinally to treat scarlet fever. Until the end of the nineteenth century, conventional doctors also used it for that purpose. Today it is one of the most commonly used homeopathic remedies among homeopaths and naturopaths for a wide variety of conditions and symptoms.

What Types of Pain Does it Help?
- Bursitis
- Cystitis
- Dysmenorrhea
- Ear infections
- Headache
- Hemorrhoids
- Neuralgia
- Osteoarthritis
- Pelvic inflammatory disease (PID)
- Rheumatoid arthritis
- Teething
- Toothache

Matching Characteristics
People who respond best to belladonna have sturdy builds, are in robust health, and have sharp, vigorous minds. When in good health they are active and charming, but when ill they become excitable and violent. Additional physical symptoms that are indications for use of belladonna and that may be alleviated by its usage include: unusual sensitivity to light, noise, touch, and pressure; hot flushed face with pale mouth and lips; and sore throat tender to the touch. Symptoms come on suddenly and usually violently.

In addition to physical ailments, mental symptoms that indicate belladonna use include restlessness, a racing imagination, feeling sleepy but being unable to sleep, hallucinations, feeling dazed and stupid, nightmares, and excited behavior.

Symptoms usually become worse with jarring motion, light, pressure, noise, exposure to the sun, eye movements, menstruation, and lying down. Pain may be worse on the right side after 11 P.M. Some relief is achieved when sitting down with the back straight, standing, staying warm, and placing warm compresses on the affected sites.

How Do You Use Belladonna?

Belladonna remedies are available in liquid, granule, powder, and tablet forms. Tablets are the most common form, but any one is equally effective when taken according to the Rule of Three. (See page 220.) See Chapter 6 for dosing instructions for children. If taking a tablet, place it under the tongue and allow it to dissolve. Alternative dosages for several specific conditions follow.

•**Bursitis:** Belladonna is indicated when the pain is worse with slight jarring motion and the joints are hot, swollen, and throbbing. Take 30c four times daily for up to seven days.

•**Cystitis (Urinary Tract Infection):** Belladonna works best when symptoms include a throbbing headache, burning pains accompanying a constant urge to urinate, dark urine, and hot burning skin. Take 6c every two hours for up to six doses, then reduce intake to three or four doses daily until symptoms begin to resolve.

•**Dysmenorrhea:** Indications for belladonna include cramps that are worse just before the period starts, a dragging sensation in the pelvic area that becomes worse when lying down, skin that is hot and flushed, and menstrual blood that is bright red. Take 30c every hour for up to 10 doses as soon as period pains begin.

•**Ear Infection:** Try belladonna when ear pain comes on suddenly, is severe, and is accompanied by a high fever. The face is usually hot and flushed and the pupils are dilated. Children may experience delirium and nightmares. Take 30c every four to six hours. If there is no improvement after three doses, try a different remedy (e.g., chamomilla or pulsatilla). Children who have a high fever and severe pain for more than 24 hours should be taken to a physician.

•**Headache:** The pain comes on suddenly and is severe. The head throbs; the face is flushed; the pupils are dilated; and the headache worsens with exposure to the sun. The hair may feel sensitive when it is brushed. The headache is usually on the right side of the head and gets worse in the afternoon and when lying down. Take 30c every 10 to 15 minutes for up to 10 doses.

•**Pelvic Inflammatory Disease (Salpingitis, PID):** The infection comes on suddenly and is accompanied by severe abdominal pain made worse by the slightest jarring. The face is bright red and burning hot. Take 30c every two hours for up to 10 doses in acute cases.

•**Teething:** When the gums are red, swollen, and throbbing and the child cries in his or her sleep, belladonna may help. Other symptoms include irritability, a flushed, hot face and glassy eyes during a fever, and a hot body without perspiration. Give 30c twice daily. If there is no improvement after two days, another remedy is needed.

•**Toothache:** The toothache comes on suddenly and is severe and throbbing. Often swelling and redness surround the affected tooth. The mouth is dry and an abscess may begin to form at the base of the hurting tooth. Take 30c every five minutes for up to 10 doses. If there is no improvement, a different remedy is needed (e.g., chamomilla, mercurius vivus).

How Does Belladonna Work?
See the explanation on page 61.

Here's the Proof
See the explanation on page 61.

Scientific investigation has revealed that belladonna contains several alkaloids, including atropine. Atropine inhibits the activity of certain nerves and relaxes smooth muscles. Whether it is responsible for any of belladonna's ability to relieve pain has not been determined scientifically.

How Safe Is Belladonna?
Warning: Because the belladonna plant is poisonous (though the homeopathic remedy is not), use only the homeopathic form of belladonna and follow your health-care provider's instructions for use.

Boswellia

What Is Boswellia?

Boswellia (*Boswellia serrata*), or frankincense, is an herb that is derived from a large tree that grows in northern Africa, India, and the Middle East. The dried resinous gum (often referred to as guggul) obtained from the tree has been valued since antiquity for its therapeutic value. The first known mention of boswellia gum was in the ancient Ayurvedic writings *Sushrita Samhita* and the *Charak Samhita*, in which the tree was said to possess the ability to give strength to the muscles. Traditional uses for boswellia include treatment of: diabetes, fever, cardiovascular conditions, skin and blood diseases, neurological problems, rheumatism, dysentery, and many other disorders.

In India, the boswellia tree is known as *shallaki*. Among certain tribes, the shallaki are regarded as sacred, ancestral property, and tribal families have guardianship over the trees to ensure they are not destroyed. The wealth of a family is determined by the number of shallaki over which it has guardianship.

What Types of Pain Does Boswellia Help?

- Back pain (lower back)
- Carpal tunnel syndrome
- Fibromyalgia
- Osteoarthritis
- Premenstrual syndrome (PMS)

- Rheumatoid arthritis
- Sciatica
- Ulcers

How Do You Use Boswellia?

Boswellia is available as a standardized extract containing 37.5 to 65 percent boswellic acids, which is the preferred form to buy. It is also available in tablet form. If purchasing a cream for topical use, look for one that has *Boswellia serrata* as the base and is standardized for boswellia acids.

•**General Dosing:** For most conditions, take 400 mg three times daily if the supplement is standardized to 37.5 percent; take 200 mg three times daily if standardized to 65 percent. For specific dosing recommendations, see below.

•**Osteoarthritis and Rheumatoid Arthritis:** Some practitioners recommend taking boswellia along with **glucosamine** (see page 128) for treatment of arthritis. Take 400 mg boswellia three times daily.

•**Premenstrual Syndrome (PMS):** For best results, choose a general dosage and combine it with 50 mg ashwaganda taken three times daily. Ashwaganda is an important herb in the Ayurvedic herbal medicine system; while not specifically a pain reliever, it enhances the anti-inflammatory activity of boswellia and contributes some diuretic properties as well.

How Does Boswellia Work?

Exactly how boswellia works is still under investigation. Beneath the bark of the boswellia lies a gummy resin, or guggul. Scientists have identified the ingredients in this gum-resin as boswellic acids. In 1992 researchers confirmed that boswellic acids are powerful inhibitors of a pro-inflammatory substance called 5-lipoxygenase. These acids, in turn, reduce production of leucotriene, an acid derivative. Simply put, boswellia acid disrupts the action of white blood cells and prevents them from rushing to the injured or traumatized site. This in turn prevents inflammation, reduces pain, and thus promotes faster healing.

Here's the Proof

Given that boswellia is an Ayurvedic remedy, most of the research had been done in India, particularly at the Regional Research Laboratory in Jammu, India. Investigators there found that boswellia extract is as effective, and in some cases even more beneficial, than the commonly used anti-inflammatory drug phenylbutazone (e.g., Azolid). Their work also shows that boswellia has no tendency to cause stomach distress or ulcers, as do conventional nonsteroidal anti-inflammatory drugs. The researchers failed to find any adverse effects to the central nervous system or cardiovascular system.

Animal studies have yielded many promising results in the treatment of pain with boswellia. In one study, for example, researchers reported that boswellia had "marked sedative and analgesic effects." The effectiveness of boswellia has been compared with other nonsteroidal anti-inflammatory drugs (NSAIDs), such as ketoprofen (e.g., Orudis). Conventional

NSAIDs disrupt the synthesis of a substance called glycosaminoglycan, a substance in the body that speeds up articular damage in people with arthritis. In one comparison, both boswellia and ketoprofen had a significant effect on glycosaminoglycan levels.

Although few studies have been done using human subjects, the results have been very encouraging. In a 1997 study, for example, one group of patients with ulcerative colitis was given boswellia extract while another group was administered the drug sulfasalazine (e.g., Azulfidine). Both groups of patients had similar improvement in pain and other symptoms, although more patients who took boswellia went into remission, and they did not suffer the side effects associated with sulfasalazine. Well-designed human studies are needed to further identify the benefits of boswellia.

How Safe Is Boswellia?
According to tests performed on healthy primates and rats, extremely high doses (1,000 mg per kilogram) of boswellia do not cause any significant changes in their blood or body chemistries. In fact, the LD-50 dose for boswellia (the dose at which 50 percent of the test subjects die) is more than 2 grams per kilogram, which is higher than that of ibuprofen (e.g., Advil, Motrin), making boswellia safer than that conventional drug.

Bromelain

What Is Bromelain?

Bromelain is a natural supplement that is not one substance but a group of sulfur-containing enzymes whose task is to digest proteins. The stem of the pineapple plant (*Ananas comusus*) is the source of this pain reliever in commercial products, although the fruit contains bromelain as well. Most of the bromelain available on the market comes from Japan, Hawaii, and Taiwan.

More than 200 scientific papers have been published about the medicinal powers of bromelain since it was first introduced as a therapeutic substance in 1957. In addition to its anti-inflammatory properties, bromelain is effective in relieving digestive disorders, enhancing wound healing, inhibiting blood platelet aggregation, and relieving sinusitis.

What Types of Pain Does Bromelain Help?

- Backache
- Carpal tunnel syndrome
- Dysmenorrhea
- Gout
- Headache
- Muscle pain
- Osteoarthritis
- Postsurgical
- Rheumatoid arthritis
- Sinusitis

- Thrombophlebitis
- Trauma

How Do You Use Bromelain?

Bromelain tablets are available in different grades, and its potency is based on one of two units of measure: milk-clotting unit (mcu) or gelatin-digesting unit (gdu). Look for products that contain 2,000 mcu per gram. At that strength, a 500-mg tablet contains 1,000 mcu activity. When treating pain and inflammation, bromelain always should be taken between meals on an empty stomach. If taken with food, the enzyme will act on the digestive process (bromelain is an excellent digestive aid) instead of the pain and inflammation.

•**General Dosing Instructions:** If you have mild to moderate pain or inflammation, take one 500-mg tablet (1,000 mcu) four times daily. For more severe conditions, take 1,500 mg (3,000 mcu) three times daily for several days, then reduce to 1,000 mg (2,000 mcu) daily. Or you can follow the specific dosages given below.

•**Back Pain:** Take 500 mg three to four times daily.

•**Carpal Tunnel Syndrome:** Take 1,000 mg twice daily during an acute attack. Reduce to 500 mg twice daily when pain and inflammation subside.

•**Gout:** During an attack, take 500 mg every three hours, then reduce to 500 mg twice daily to help prevent additional attacks.

•**Rheumatoid Arthritis and Muscle Pain:** Take 500 to 750 mg (1,800 to 2,000 mcu) three times daily.

•**Postoperative Pain:** Take 500 mg three times daily.

•**Thrombophlebitis:** For relief of pain, swelling, and tenderness, a course of 400 to 800 mg daily, when taken as a complement to a conventional analgesic, may provide additional relief. Consult with your healthcare provider before starting treatment with bromelain.

How Does Bromelain Work?

Bromelain scores many points as a pain reliever, especially as an anti-inflammatory agent, but it also prevents swelling, relaxes muscles, prevents ulcers, and promotes wound healing. Bromelain's anti-inflammatory effects appear to be related to several actions. One is its ability to break down fibrin, a protein that promotes inflammation by blocking blood vessels and causing a buildup of fluid in tissue. Fibrin also is active in the formation of blood clots.

Bromelain also has the ability to inhibit the production of kinins, factors that cause inflammation, swelling, and pain and that are particularly active in sports and other traumatic injuries. In addition to its pain-fighting activities, bromelain is also an effective antibiotic in certain infectious conditions (e.g., bronchitis, pneumonia) and may have anti-cancer effects.

Here's the Proof

The excellent results from the clinical studies that have been done with bromelain have prompted more widespread use of this pineapple derivative. A report in the February 1998 *Nutrition Science News,* for example, notes that bromelain has been successful in treating sports injuries, arthritis, and postsurgical swelling. A study reported in 1995 of 59 patients who had suffered blunt injuries showed that the patients got significant relief of pain and swelling when using bromelain. Studies among people undergoing oral surgery show bromelain significantly reduces swelling and duration of pain when compared with a placebo. Similar results are experienced by women who take bromelain both before and after episiotomy.

Among people with sports injuries, a study conducted in 1960 demonstrated impressive results. Of 74 boxers who took bromelain after a fight, in 58 of them bruising cleared completely within four days. Among the 72 controls, only 10 had complete healing within the same period.

Several studies show that bromelain is effective in reducing the pain, tenderness, and swelling that accompany inflammation of the veins (thrombophlebitis) when it is given in conjunction with analgesics. Researchers found that doses of 400 to 800 mg provide effective, consistent relief.

How Safe Is Bromelain?
Bromelain causes no side effects for the majority of people, even at dosages as high as 2 grams daily. Rare cases of nausea, vomiting, diarrhea, and rash have been reported. Among sensitive individuals, allergic reactions are possible. Do not take bromelain if you are pregnant, have a blood-clotting disorder, have ulcers, or are taking blood thinning drugs (e.g., warfarin, enoxaparin).

Bryonia

What Is Bryonia?

The homeopathic remedy bryonia (*Bryonia alba*) is derived from a perennial climbing vine that grows wild in southern Europe in woods and vineyards and is cultivated in the United States. Another species, *Bryonia diocia*, is used to make the homeopathic remedy as well. Bryonia is also known as wild bryony, white bryony, and wild hops. The plant has long-branched, spindle-shaped roots that have an unpleasant taste and odor that disappear when dried. The tincture is made from the fresh root before the plant flowers in early spring (flowers are greenish yellow) or from the whole fresh plant.

The medicinal value of bryonia was known to the ancient Greeks, who used the root as a purgative (a substance that causes vomiting). It is believed the Greeks gave the plant its name, derived from *bryo*, meaning "to thrust or sprout," a reference to the speed with which the vine grows. Accidental ingestion of the root can cause tissue inflammation, severe vomiting, and violent diarrhea, all symptoms that the homeopathic version can ease.

Dr. Samuel Hahnemann recognized the many benefits of bryonia early in his research and used it to treat cholera, typhus, rheumatic conditions, headache, and neuralgias. Unlike belladonna, bryonia is best used in conditions that develop slowly, such as rheumatoid arthritis and other arthritic disorders.

What Types of Pain Does Bryonia Help?
- Backache
- Colic
- Fibromyalgia
- Headache (acute)
- Neuralgias
- Rheumatoid arthritis
- Toothache

Matching Characteristics
Among infants and children, characteristics that indicate bryonia use include sensitivity to light and noise, dislike of being carried or touched, irritability, and increased thirst for cold drinks. Adult patients tend to be sluggish with poor circulation, have a dark complexion and dark hair, are easily irritated or angered, and are methodical. They are often accountants or involved in the insurance or banking industries and are prudent and calculating. Their pains come and go and eventually become continuous and are worse from motion, heat, and stuffy rooms. Mental conditions alleviated include irritability, dullness, complete stupefaction (in severe cases), and hopelessness. Patients often worry about money, their job, and the future. Mental symptoms improve with cool fresh air.

Physical symptoms that improve with bryonia include violent headaches that often are worsened by slight movement, too much food or alcohol; colds and coughing that are relieved by application of firm pressure and cold compresses; stabbing pains in the eyes;

dry, sore lips; pain in the rib cage made worse by coughing, drinking, and warm rooms; cold hands and feet; in rheumatism sufferers, hot swollen painful joints made worse by cold drafts and slight movement; inflammation of the membranes of the brain and spinal cord; and dizziness.

How Do You Use Bryonia?

Bryonia remedies are available in tincture, granule, powder, and tablet forms. Tablets are the most common form, but any one is equally effective when taken according to the Rule of Three (see page 220.)

If taking a tablet, place it under the tongue and allow it to dissolve. See Chapter 6 for dosing instructions for children.

Alternative dosages for several specific conditions follow.

•**Back Pain (Lower Back):** Bryonia is helpful for back pain caused by overexertion. The pain typically appears in cold, dry weather and is worse with the slightest movement. The back feels bruised and is very sensitive to touch. Take 6c four times daily for up to 10 days.

•**Bursitis:** The pain worsens with heat or the slightest movement. Take 30c four times a day for up to seven days.

•**Colic:** The child prefers to lie very still because movement makes the pain worse. Doubling over and warmth bring some relief. If using the 30c formulation, give two to three times daily until improvement occurs. If using the 6c formulation, give one dose every hour for up to six doses, then reduce frequency when improvement occurs.

•**Fibromyalgia:** This pain, in the neck, limbs, and back, is worse with movement and when there are dry, cold east winds. Pain improves when pressure is applied to the affected sites. Take 30c every three hours for up to two days.

•**Headache:** Indicated for splitting or bursting head pain that gets worse with the slightest motion, noise, light, and eye movement. Patients best suited for bryonia are very irritable and like to be left alone.

•**Rheumatoid Arthritis:** This remedy can help those who experience greater pain with small movements and with the arrival of cold, dry weather and less pain when pressure is applied to the affected sites. Take 6c four times daily for up to two weeks.

•**Toothache:** Bryonia is indicated when the teeth feel too long; when movement and hot food and drinks make the pain worse; when the pain is alleviated by lying down on the painful side; and when the affected area is pressed. Take 30c every five minutes for up to 10 doses.

How Does Bryonia Work?
See the explanation on page 61.

Bryonia contains a resin called bryoresin, which is believed to be the source of the plant's activity. Bryoresin acts on the fibrous tissues and ligaments around joints, which become inflamed and painful with rheumatism.

Here's the Proof
See the explanation on page 61.

How Safe Is Bryonia?
See explanation on page 64.

Calcarea Carbonica

What Is Calcarea Carbonica?
Calcarea carbonica, or calcium carbonate, is also known as calcarea ostrearum. It is derived from the natural secretions of the European oyster, *Ostrea edulis*. This homeopathic remedy is prepared from the layer of crystals of calcium carbonate that are located in the middle layer of the oyster's shell. Traditionally it has been used to treat symptoms of exhaustion, depression, and anxiety.

What Types of Pain Does Calcarea Carbonica Help?
• Back pain (lower)
• Ear infections (chronic)
• Headache
• Muscle pain
• Osteoarthritis
• Premenstrual syndrome (PMS)
• Rheumatoid arthritis
• Teething
• Toothache
• Trauma (fractures slow to heal)

Matching Characteristics

Adults who respond well to calcarea carbonica are usually fair, flabby, and overweight. The psychological profile tends to include people who are stubborn and indecisive and those who find mental effort to be exhausting and nearly impossible. Children who benefit from the remedy have coarse skin and curly hair, tend to be chubby and clumsy, and have a chalky pale complexion. Some are prone to experience head sweats at night.

Accompanying physical symptoms that indicate calcarea carbonica use include cataracts; swollen tonsils, lymph nodes, and adenoids, copious perspiration; aversion to meat, coffee, and milk; feeling better when constipated; and craving pickles, eggs, and sweets. Emotional and mental symptoms include depression, emotional fragility, fear of making a fool of oneself, fear of the dark, bouts of workaholism followed by sudden laziness, resentment, preoccupation with trivia, poor memory, brooding over little details, and forgetting what one has just read.

Conditions that make symptoms worse include drafts, exertion, and cold damp wind. Improvement comes when the person is constipated or is lying on the affected side.

How Do You Use Calcarea Carbonica?

Calcarea carbonica remedies are available in tincture, granule, powder, and tablet forms. Tablets are the most common form, but any one is equally effective when taken according to the Rule of Three. (See page 220.) If taking a tablet, place it under the tongue and allow it to dissolve. See Chapter 6 for dosing instructions for children. Alternative dosing suggestions for several specific conditions follow.

•**Premenstrual Syndrome (PMS):** Symptoms include lack of energy, clumsiness, cold sweats, swollen painful breasts, tiredness, and a craving for sweets. Take 30c every 12 hours for up to three days, starting 24 hours before PMS symptoms are due.

•**Teething:** Calcarea carbonica is indicated for infants who have delayed teething.

•**Toothache:** Indicated for toothache that occurs when you eat; when exposure to cold air and cold drinks makes the pain worse, especially if you are pregnant. Take 6c every 5 minutes for up to 10 doses.

How Does Calcarea Carbonica Work?
One theory as to why calcarea carbonica works is that it rebalances the body's calcium levels. Another is that it corrects dysfunctions in calcium metabolism. The validity of these explanations has not been proven scientifically. For additional details, see page 61.

Here's the Proof
See the explanation on page 61.

How Safe Is Calcarea Carbonica?
See the explanation on page 64.

Calcarea Phosphorica

What Is Calcarea Phosphorica?

Calcarea phosphorica, or calcium phosphate, is made by adding dilute phosphoric acid to lime water. This homeopathic remedy often is prescribed for children who are experiencing growing pains, headache, teething, and other painful conditions. Calcium phosphate is essential to growth and maintenance of blood cells and connective tissue. One obvious homeopathic use is to accelerate healing of bone fractures.

What Types of Pain Does Calcarea Phosphorica Help?

- Backache
- Dysmenorrhea (menstrual cramps)
- Growing pains
- Headache
- Osteoarthritis
- Trauma (broken bones)

Matching Characteristics

Calcarea phosphorica suits people who are discontented and uncertain about what they want. They are usually thin with dark hair, long legs, and a sagging abdomen. As babies they were late in walking. Among children, calcarea phosphorica works best for those who are or were slow to teethe or who have gone through a growth spurt and have become exhausted and pale.

Mental symptoms alleviated include nervousness, restlessness, fidgeting, and a dislike of routine; need for stimulation; and difficulty getting up in the morning. Physical symptoms that indicate this remedy include painful bones and joints, growing pains, fractures slow to heal, and headaches in children. Symptoms are aggravated by damp, cold, changeable weather; exertion; lifting things; worrying; grief; and sexual excesses. Summer and warm dry weather often produce dramatic improvement.

How Do You Use Calcarea Phosphorica?

Calcarea phosphorica remedies are available in tincture, granule, powder, and tablet forms. Tablets are the most common form, but any one is equally effective when taken according to the Rule of Three. (See page 220.) If taking a tablet, place it under the tongue and allow it to dissolve. See Chapter 6 for dosing instructions for children.

Take calcarea phosphorica according to the Rule of Three for the conditions mentioned above. If you have osteoarthritis, calcarea phosphorica is beneficial for flare-ups only, not for chronic pain. Take 6c four times daily for up to two weeks if the affected joints feel cold and numb, you have an increase in pain and stiffness when the weather changes, and you experience weakness when climbing stairs.

How Does Calcarea Phosphorica Work?

See the explanation on page 61.

Here's the Proof
See the explanation on page 61.

How Safe Is Calcarea Phosphorica?
See the explanation on page 64.

Cayenne (Capsaicin)

What Is Cayenne?
Cayenne pepper is the fruit (technically a berry) of a tropical shrub called *Capsicum annuum*. Also known as red hot pepper and chili pepper, it is a native of tropical America but is now grown in other parts of the world, especially Mexico, China, southeast Asia, and Italy. The peppers were named by Spanish explorers who, along with Columbus, were searching for peppercorns like those that grow in India. Apparently the explorers thought the cayenne pepper flavor was similar to that of peppercorns. When brought back to Europe, the peppers quickly became popular as a food and spice.

According to folk medicine tales, cayenne has been used for hundreds of years to treat fever, sore throats, asthma, digestive problems, and various respiratory infections. The primary active healing ingredient in cayenne is capsaicin, which is also responsible for making the pepper hot. Paradoxically, however, although cayenne is hot to the taste, it actually reduces body temperature by stimulating the area of the hypothalamus responsible for temperature control. Other chemicals in cayenne pepper include apsaicine, capsacutin, capsanthine, and capsico. Cayenne also contains a significant amount of vitamins A and B, folic acid, and carotenoids, and has more vitamin C than an orange.

What Types of Pain Does Cayenne Help?
- Cluster headache
- Diabetic neuropathy
- Muscle pain
- Osteoarthritis
- Postsurgical (especially postmastectomy)
- Rheumatoid arthritis
- Shingles
- Trigeminal neuralgia

How Do You Use Cayenne?
Cayenne is available as a cream or ointment for topical use; in tablet, capsule, softgel, tincture, liquid, and fresh or dried herb form for internal use; and as a spray. Creams and ointments are used for pain relief, while the other forms, except for the spray, are for digestive disorders. Purchase a cream or ointment that contains 0.025 to 0.075 percent capsaicin.

Apply a thin coat over the affected area at least three to four times a day and rub it in thoroughly. Wear disposable gloves or wash your hands with warm soapy water after you handle cayenne and avoid touching your eyes, nose, or contact lenses. If you are treating your hands for pain, keep the cayenne on for

30 minutes before you wash it off, to allow the cream to penetrate your skin. It may take one or more weeks before you experience significant pain relief.

Although your doctor can write a prescription for capsaicin cream, many over-the-counter brands are equally as effective and likely cost much less. If you suffer from cluster headache, cayenne spray has proven effective. The spray should be used only under a doctor's supervision.

How Does Cayenne Work?

A neurotransmitter called substance P is responsible for transmitting pain signals from the periphery of the body to the brain. Capsaicin works two ways against substance P. Repeated applications of capsaicin cream to the skin or mucous membranes depletes the pain fibers of substance P, thus blocking pain signals. Capsaicin also inhibits the body's production of substance P. Because capsaicin affects only a specific type of neuron in the skin, it is well suited to treat arthritis, fibromyalgia, diabetic neuropathy, shingles, and other types of chronic pain that can be treated with a topical remedy.

Here's the Proof

Cayenne is one of the few herbs that has undergone extensive testing for the treatment of pain, so much so that it has won Food and Drug Administration (FDA) approval for use in postherpetic neuralgia (shingles) and is a key ingredient in several over-the-counter and prescription lotions and creams.

Use of cayenne for shingles has been especially impressive. Of the dozens of studies conducted, the general results are that about 50 percent of people with postherpetic neuralgia get significant improvement when using a topical cream containing 0.025 percent capsaicin and up to 75 percent respond favorably when the 0.075 percent cream is used. On average, patients note substantial relief after two weeks of treatment.

Studies of topically applied capsaicin cream for patients with arthritis demonstrate good results. In a double-blind study conducted by Chad Deal, M.D., of Case Western Reserve University in Cleveland, 80 percent of patients treated with 0.025 percent capsaicin cream had up to a 50 percent reduction in pain after only two weeks, although those with rheumatoid arthritis reported better results than those with osteoarthritis. Patients in the placebo group experienced no relief. In another study, reported in a 1992 edition of the *Journal of Rheumatology*, the opposite was true: Patients with osteoarthritis reported better results.

Patients who suffer with debilitating cluster headaches experience significantly less severe pain when using a capsaicin nasal spray, according to results of double-blind studies. The spray reduces both the number and severity of clusters and in some cases can even eliminate the symptoms. This finding is particularly important because few remedies, conventional or complementary, have any impact on cluster headache pain. Because capsaicin is very irritating to the mucous membranes, the spray should be used under a doctor's supervision only.

Another condition highly resistant to treatment is trigeminal neuralgia. Although only a few studies using capsaicin to treat this condition exist, the results are promising. In a study reported in 1992, for example, 10 of 12 patients who used capsaicin three times a day for several days reported complete or partial relief from pain. After four of the patients relapsed, they underwent another round of treatment; thereafter none experienced a recurrence.

Numerous studies involving hundreds of patients with diabetic neuropathy show that the majority of individuals who use topical capsaicin experience improvement. In one multicenter, double-blind study involving 252 patients, half were given capsaicin cream and half a placebo (an inert cream). By the end of the eight-week study, 74 percent of the patients who received capsaicin had significant pain relief. In another study conducted at the University of Vermont, 90 percent of patients treated with capsaicin cream reported excellent results.

Similar results are reported from women who were given capsaicin cream following breast reconstruction or mastectomy, both of which are associated with much pain. Pain relief was significant when patients used the cream four times daily for four to six weeks.

How Safe Is Capsaicin?
Topical application can cause a burning sensation that ranges from mild to intolerable in a very few cases.

You should test to see if you are overly sensitive to capsaicin before using it freely. Apply capsaicin lotion or cream to a small painful spot several times a day for one to two days. If you do not experience any significant discomfort (a mild burning or warm feeling is common for the first few days after starting capsaicin), then you can enlarge the area treated. The nasal spray should be used only under direct medical supervision.

Chinese Herbs

What Are Chinese Herbs?
Traditional Chinese herbal medicine is based on a complex system of diagnosis that aims to restore harmony and balance to the body's energy, also known as *chi*, or vital energy. According to practitioners of traditional Chinese medicine, disease and other disorders are caused by disturbances in the flow of chi, or by an imbalance between yin and yang, the complementary states of being. Chinese herbal formulas are designed to restore the flow and the balance.

Chinese medicine practitioners use herbal combinations or formulas much more often than single herbs to get the desired effect. Herbs are divided into four categories according to their ability to strengthen or supplement the body, circulate or disperse chi and the body's fluids, redistribute or consolidate chi or bodily fluids, and purge and eliminate blockages and toxins. A Chinese medicine practitioner selects herbs

based on the patient's state of harmony and dishar-
mony—the balance of his or her yin and yang. Individual herbs are categorized by many criteria, a few
of which include their energy (hot, warm, neutral,
cool, or cold); taste (pungent, mildly sweet, bland,
sour, bitter, or salty); whether they are yang, yin, or
neutral; and their action (i.e., how the herb affects the
body and the specific organs).

In Chinese medicine, illnesses also are assigned
their own special energy and other characteristics. Illnesses can be either hot or cold, damp or dry. Addi-
tionally they are defined as being either internal
(conditions that affect the inside of the body) or external (those that affect the skin, throat, or muscles,
such as chills, sweating, fever, and body aches).
These two categories are combined to further help
define disease; for example, a person can have signs
of external heat or internal damp. High fever is an
example of external heat; nausea an example of internal damp. An illness also is classified according to
whether it is one of deficiency (e.g., lack of blood as
in anemia) or excess (too much heat, as with fever).
Unlike conventional medicine, which has an overall
treatment approach to disease and ailments, Chinese
medicine recognizes that each illness and the person
it is affecting have their own special energy. Two
women, each with a throbbing headache, would likely
receive the same medication if they went to a conventional medical doctor. Chinese medicine practitioners, however, would base their prescription on the
energy of the illness and the individual; they would

treat the imbalances that underlie the symptoms displayed by the patient, not the symptoms themselves. Thus they would look at the two women who had a throbbing headache: one is tall with a rapid pulse and a coated tongue and the other is short with a shallow pulse and a dry tongue. Because they have different physical characteristics and distinct conditions that must be balanced, each woman would receive a different herbal combination, even though a throbbing headache is the primary complaint of both.

What Types of Pain Do Chinese Herbs Help?

Traditional Chinese medicine states that disease and illness occur when chi is disturbed. Disturbance can be caused by external forces, internal forces, or incidents such as accidents, lifestyle habits, and injuries. Although Chinese herbal formulas can address every type of pain covered in this book, our discussion is limited to the most common, effective, and readily available herbal combinations, including remedies for:

- Backache
- Childbirth
- Dysmenorrhea
- Headache
- Hemorrhoids
- Migraine
- Muscle pain
- Osteoarthritis
- Premenstrual syndrome (PMS)
- Rheumatoid arthritis

- Sciatica
- Sinusitis
- Toothache

How Do You Use Chinese Herbs?

Chinese herbal medicine is a complex yet effective option for pain relief. To meet the growing demand for Chinese herbal remedies, some formulas are now available already prepared, in capsule, tablet, decoction, or powder forms. Such formulas may not fit your situation exactly, because Chinese herbal remedies are often "built" from a base remedy, to which are added complementary herbs to balance a specific individual's specific needs. However, they contain a balanced combination of herbs that have proven to be the most effective overall and often will provide good results. Unless you are familiar with Chinese herbal remedies, it is best to consult a knowledgeable Chinese medicine practitioner or herbalist to help you choose the best herbal remedy for you or to perhaps mix one for you.

Whether you choose your own Chinese herbal remedies or not, it is useful to know which are the most helpful in the treatment of pain. The following is a brief description of a few of the herbs used most often to treat pain as well as those you are likely to find in ready-made formulas.

•**Aconite (Fu Zi)** is the hottest herb in Chinese medicine. It is indicated for severe pain, arthritis (especially in the lower limbs), sciatica, lower back pain, neuralgia, and abdominal pain. It is often combined with cinnamon bark, ginger, ginseng, and atractylodes (a Chinese herb). Aconite is also a homeopathic remedy.

•**Angelica Root (Du Huo)** is indicated for joint pain that increases with cold and diminishes with heat; head pain in which the head feels heavy; toothache; and back pain accompanied by difficulty in rotating or bending the trunk.

•**Bupleurum (Chai Hu)** relieves hemorrhoids, PMS, and menstrual difficulties.

•**Cinnamon Twig (Gui Zhi)** is an anti-inflammatory and is used to treat muscle pain. Cinnamon is an ingredient in many pain-relieving formulas.

•**Corydalis (Yan Hu Suo)** is considered to be the most effective painkiller in traditional Chinese medicine. It raises the pain threshold and is a potent analgesic and anti-inflammatory. Often it is the main ingredient in formulas used to treat dysmenorrhea, headache, arthritis, sinusitis, and toothache. It is sometimes mixed with cinnamon to treat menstrual pain. A corydalis decoction, which is prepared using a special process, relieves pain and bruising from injuries.

•**Dong Quai (Tang Kuei)** is helpful for dysmenorrhea, PMS, muscle pain, and sciatica. It improves blood flow and regulates uterine contractions; some researchers believe this action is the basis of its benefit for dysmenorrhea.

•**Ligusticum (Chuan Xiong),** also known as privet

fruit or Japanese wax privet, is used to treat menstrual pain, painful labor, headache, and migraine. It is often combined with dong quai for treatment of menstrual pain.

•**Notopterygium (Qiang Huo)** helps relieve headache and back pain accompanied by difficulty in rotating or bending the trunk.

•**Pueraria (Ge Gen),** also known as **kudzu** or kuzu root, is beneficial for those with headache or muscle aches and pains. It has a bland, chalky taste and is often mixed with ginger, licorice, or cinnamon, or with fruit and other ingredients for a delicious beverage. (See pages 102–103 for recipes.) It relieves muscle pain by neutralizing acidity in the body.

•**Rehmannia (Di Huang)** is a common ingredient in formulas that treat arthritis, back pain, hemorrhoids, menstrual pain, and sciatica. It is an anti-inflammatory and sometimes is combined with bupleurum to treat autoimmune conditions such as fibromyalgia and rheumatoid arthritis.

You can find some of the following preblended commercial products in Chinese pharmacies, listed in catalogs or through mail order or on the Internet. Ask a knowledgeable professional to help you make your selection.

•**AC-Q:** This remedy is sold as a tablet and consists of a long list of herbs that help ease the pain, fatigue, and other symptoms associated with fibromyalgia.

•**Ba Wei Di Huang Wan:** Also sometimes known as Eight-Ingredient Pill with Rehmannia. The main ingredient is rehmannia, and it is indicated for back pain and sciatica.

•**Du Huo Ji Sheng Tang:** This remedy can be purchased as a tea. Its primary ingredient is angelica root (du huo), with lesser amounts of cinnamon bark, ligusticum, ginseng, and 11 other herbs, and it is used to treat arthritis, sciatica, and back pain.

•**Peppermint:** Apply several drops of peppermint juice into the ears to relieve earache.

•**Shu Jing Huo Xue Tang:** Available as the commercial product called Mobility 2, it is based on an ancient remedy that reduces the pain and inflammation of arthritis and related disorders.

•**Si Wu Tang:** Also called Four Substance Decoction, this remedy relieves menstrual pain. It consists of rehmannia, peony, angelica, and ligusticum.

•**Yan Hu Suo Zhi Tang Pian:** Conditions that may respond to this remedy include arthritis, headache, sinusitis, and toothache. Corydalis, turmeric (jiang huang), and myrrh are three of the main ingredients.

KUDZU RECIPES

Here are some delicious ways to take your medicine! Each recipe supplies 3 g kudzu (pueraria) which is one-quarter to one-half the usual daily dose prescribed in Chinese medicine.

PINK KUDZU (makes 2 cups)
1 teaspoon (6 g) ground or crushed kudzu
½ cup soy milk
1 pint strawberries

¼ cup nonfat soy yogurt
2 teaspoons balsamic vinegar
1 tablespoon maple syrup

Whisk the kudzu into the soy milk and set aside. In a food processor, combine the remaining ingredients and process until smooth. Pour in the kudzu mixture and process again. Serve chilled.

PEACH GRAPEFRUIT BLIZZARD (makes 2 cups)
1 teaspoon (6 g) ground or crushed kudzu
⅓ cup seltzer water
2 ripe pitted peaches, peeled and cut into chunks
¼ cup fresh lemon juice
¼ cup soy milk
½ cup fresh grapefruit juice

Whisk the kudzu into the seltzer water, then set aside. Combine the remaining ingredients in a food processor and process until smooth. Pour in the kudzu mixture and process again. Serve over crushed ice.

How Do Chinese Herbs Work?

The system of Chinese herbal medicine is too complex to be explained here fully. Briefly, the Chinese believe plants heal because they are part of an intimate network in which everything in the universe has both a yin and yang component, opposing yet complementary forces existing within each person and thing. Thus herbs that possess certain yin-yang properties are matched with the yin-yang state of the person who is in need of balancing and with the properties and energy of the illness. A person with arthritis pain that is accompanied by chills, headache, dizziness, and a white greasy coating on the tongue may be given a warming herb (e.g., cinnamon, or gui zhi) along with herbs to unblock the flow of yang chi to resolve the other symptoms (e.g., ephedra, aconite, angelica).

Health is a state of balance between yin and yang. When the right herbs are chosen, they can restore that balance. Dr. Fung Fung explains that empirical knowledge and practical experience has been the basis of the herbal formulas he has prescribed for 60 years. Given that herbs are Nature's gifts "which nourish and sustain life," and we are part of Nature, "we will appreciate the value of nature's products, and will not hesitate to take advantage of these products."

Here's the Proof
Chinese herbal formulas have withstood the ultimate test: the test of time. For approximately 3,000 years, the formulas have been tested, reformulated, and retested by hundreds of millions of Chinese people and now, as Chinese medicine has grown in popularity in the West, by Western people as well. Some scientifically conducted studies have been done by researchers in Asia, Europe, and the United States, but they have largely been confined to single herbs, such as ginseng and licorice, rather than using the complex combinations typical of Chinese herbal medicine.

Dr. Fung Fung, author of *Sixty Years in Search of Cures: An Herbalist's Success with Chinese Herbs,* notes "that herbs are still widely used is testimony to their safety and effectiveness." In light of his 60 years of experience and the vast history of Chinese herbal medicine, he says that "an effective prescription depends more on the medicinal effects of the herbs than it does on medical theory."

How Safe Is Chinese Herbal Medicine?

Chinese herbal remedies are safe when taken as directed. Because Chinese herbal formulas can be very potent, it is recommended that you not self-diagnosis or take a remedy without the assistance of a person knowledgeable in Chinese herbal medicine. Some Chinese herbal formulas have significant side effects or contraindications, as do some Western herbal remedies.

Colocynthis

What Is Colocynthis?

Colocynthis (*Citrullus colocynthus*) is a plant with a hairy stem and yellow flowers that thrives in sandy soil in hot, dry climates. It is also referred to as bitter cucumber and bitter apple, although its fruit is yellow and as large as an orange. The pulp contains a strong poison that acts on the bowels, causing extreme pain and straining during defecation. The homeopathic remedy, which is made by drying the fruit and grinding it into a powder, is nontoxic.

What Types of Pain Does Colocynthis Help?
- Colic
- Dysmenorrhea (menstrual cramps)
- Gout
- Headache
- Rheumatoid arthritis
- Sciatica
- Trigeminal neuralgia

Matching Characteristics
Individuals who are most likely to benefit from taking colocynthis have fair skin and light hair. Mental and emotional symptoms associated with use of colocynthis include anger and indignation, extreme irritability, and embarrassment caused by offensive remarks. Conditions that indicate use of colocynthis include headaches that improve by applying warmth or pressure; trigeminal neuralgia; stomach pain with nausea and vomiting; shooting nerve pain in the kidney area; sciatica; gout; rheumatism; agonizing abdominal pain alleviated by lying on the side with knees drawn up to the chin; and spasmodic abdominal pain with diarrhea. All symptoms are made worse when you are angry, eating, drinking, or exposed to damp cold. They improve with firm pressure, warmth, sleep, coffee, and passing wind.

How Do You Use Colocynthis?
Colocynthis remedies are available in tincture, granule, powder, and tablet forms. Tablets are the most

common form, but any one is equally effective when taken according to the Rule of Three. (See page 220.) Alternative dosages and characteristics for several specific conditions follow.

If taking a tablet, place it under the tongue and allow it to dissolve. See Chapter 6 for dosing instructions for children

•**Colic:** Colocynthis can be beneficial in children who are extremely irritable, who twist and cry angrily, and who have cramping pains that cause them to double over. Diarrhea also may be present. Pressure on the abdomen and warmth relieve the pain. If a child has these characteristics, give 30c two to three times daily until improvement occurs. Dissolve the powder in 4 ounces distilled or boiled water and give to the child by teaspoon or in a bottle. Do not mix the remedy with formula or juice.

•**Dysmenorrhea:** Colocynthis works best for severe menstrual cramps that are relieved when you bend over or apply heat or pressure.

•**Gout:** Colocynthis may be effective when the pain is relieved by heat or pressure.

•**Headache:** Try colocynthis when the headache is on the left side and has spread to the ear, and when it is worse with touch.

•**Sciatica:** Colocynthis is especially useful for sciatica experienced as a cramping pain in the hip, usually on the right side, and which is relieved by lying on the pain and applying heat.

How Does Colocynthis Work?
See the explanation on page 61.

Here's the Proof
See the explanation on page 61.

How Safe Is Colocynthis?
See the explanation on page 64.

Devil's Claw

What Is Devil's Claw?
Devil's claw (*Harpagophytum procumbens*) is an herb that derives its name from the clawlike shape of its seed pods, which are about the size of an adult's hand. The English call it grapple plant or wood spider. The plant belongs to the *Pedaliaceae* family and is found in southwest Africa, primarily in the Kalahari, where it creeps along the ground. When the rains come, its fragile stems produce trumpet-shaped flowers. To survive the long droughts typical of the desert region in which it grows, devil's claw has long roots—up to three feet in length—which produce brown tubers at various levels. These tubers, which store water and absorb trace minerals, are used to make the herbal remedy.

Devil's claw became popular among Europeans early in the 20th century after a German farmer named G. H. Mehnert heard about its healing properties. Mehnert gathered some of the plants while he was traveling in Africa; upon his return to Germany, he told the medical community about his find. The herb then became the subject of much study to discover if the claims of the African natives were true.

African natives have long used devil's claw to treat arthritis, rheumatism, malaria, menstrual problems, headache, and digestive disorders. Traditionally the natives use the dried root to make a tea for internal problems and prepare the fresh root as an ointment to treat skin disorders. In Chinese medicine, devil's claw is regarded as a remedy for an ailing heart and blood circulation. The plant caught the attention of a German scientist, who discovered that it has many of the same chemical properties as phenylbutazone, a conventional drug used to treat arthritis.

What Types of Pain Does Devil's Claw Help?
- Back pain (low) from spondylosis
- Dysmenorrhea
- Gallbladder disorders
- Gout
- Headache
- Liver disorders
- Neuralgia
- Osteoarthritis
- Rheumatoid arthritis

How Do You Use Devil's Claw?
Devil's claw is available in bulk as fresh root or powder, tincture, dry solid extract, and in capsule form.

When purchasing devil's claw, look for a product that contains ground fresh roots, not sun-dried roots, because oxidation causes the roots to lose their potency. To prepare a decoction, add ½ to 1 teaspoon ground devil's claw powder to 1 cup boiling water. Simmer covered for 15 minutes, strain, and discard herb pieces. The general standard dosage of devil's claw is 3 cups per day of the decoction or 20 drops tincture in water twice daily. To begin treatment with devil's claw, take the recommended dosage for three weeks, then stop for one week. Begin again, alternating treatment every other week: one week on, one week off. This pattern can continue as long as you need treatment.

•**Dysmenorrhea.** Use of devil's claw for menstrual cramps is largely anecdotal, yet it is so safe, it's worth a try. Begin with tincture or decoction.

•**Gout and Osteoarthritis.** Three times a day take: 1 to 2 g dried powdered root; *or* 4 to 5 milliliters (ml) tincture; *or* 400 mg dry solid extract. Devil's claw can be injected around affected joints in people who have arthritis.

How Does Devil's Claw Work?
Devil's claw contains more than 40 constituents, yet scientists believe the three main glycosides—harpagide, harpagoside, and procumbide—are responsible for much of the plant's ability to relieve pain and inflammation. These glycosides are found in both the main and secondary tubers, but the secondary tubers contain about twice as much of these substances.

Studies conducted at the University of Jena in Germany in 1958 revealed that devil's claw has anti-inflammatory properties comparable to those of cortisone and phenylbutazone, yet it does not have the side effects associated with these conventional drugs. Subsequent studies conducted in other countries have since verified these findings.

Here's the Proof

Studies of devil's claw as an anti-inflammatory and pain reliever for osteoarthritis have been largely limited to animals and have produced conflicting results. Some pharmacological research indicates that devil's claw is as effective as the anti-inflammatory and analgesic drug phenylbutazone; others suggest it has little value in these areas. These inconsistencies are believed to be related to a lack of standardization of the formulas used in the studies.

A French study published in the medical journal *Medecine Actuelle* reported that 89 percent of 43 patients with osteoarthritis had reduced pain and 84 percent had increased range of motion after 60 days of treatment with devil's claw. Many of the patients experienced results in as little as eight days. In a Germany study 80 percent of those receiving devil's claw had improved pain relief compared with 72 percent of those taking phenylbutazone. Although the difference in relief was not great, devil's claw did not cause any of the side effects or intolerances experienced by those who took phenylbutazone.

In 1994 a report in the *Canadian Journal of Phys-*

iology and Pharmacology indicated that devil's claw extract injected near arthritic joints is effective. This practice is used in Germany to ease swelling and pain but has not yet been embraced in the United States.

Despite the lack of convincing scientific evidence, many herbalists continue to prescribe devil's claw infusions for inflammation. For now, anecdotal reports of its effectiveness appear to support its widespread use.

How Safe Is Devil's Claw?
Devil's claw has not undergone a great deal of investigation, yet side effects in humans thus far have been rare. The few reported include ringing in the ears, headache, and loss of appetite. Diabetics may notice a rise in blood sugar levels, and individuals with gallstones, heart disorders, or ulcers should ask their physician before taking devil's claw. Information about how it interacts with conventional medications is scarce.

Feverfew

What Is Feverfew?
This member of the same family (*Asteraceae*) that includes the black-eyed susan, marigold, echinacea, sunflower, and artichoke grows throughout the United States and Europe. Several stories exist as to how feverfew (*Tanacetum parthenium*) got its name. One is that it is a variation on the Latin word *febri-*

fugia, which means "to drive out fever." This explanation has been challenged, however, by scholars who note that ancient physicians called the plant *parthenium* and dispensed it to patients for menstrual disorders and melancholy. During the Middle Ages, it was renamed *featherfoil* because the plant has feathery leaves. Eventually the word became *featherfew* and finally feverfew. Despite its name, feverfew has no apparent ability to reduce fever.

Throughout the centuries, feverfew has been best known for the treatment of migraine, arthritis, earache, dysmenorrhea, and intestinal parasites. Because of its strong odor, especially when crushed, herbalists of centuries past planted the herb around their homes to ward off malaria, which people used to believe was caused by bad air. (*Mala* is Italian for "bad.")

What Types of Pain Does Feverfew Help?
• Migraine
• Rheumatoid arthritis

How Do You Use Feverfew?
Feverfew is available in capsule, liquid extract, and tablet form and as fresh, freeze-dried, or heat-dried leaves. Feverfew is effective only if it contains sufficient levels of parthenolide, preferably 0.4 to 0.66 percent (approximately 500 to 800 mcg parthenolide). At that level, a dosage of 250 to 400 mg feverfew twice daily is generally enough to prevent migraine, while 1 to 2 g may be needed during an attack. If you prefer the liquid leaf extract, take 4 to 8 ml up to three times daily.

The best form of feverfew to buy is one that is produced with as little heat as possible, as parthenolide loses much of its potency when heated. Eating the fresh leaves can be both effective and inexpensive, especially if you grow your own. Drawbacks to eating feverfew are its bitter taste and its tendency to cause mouth irritation in some people. To help remedy both of these problems, eat two to three leaves daily on a sandwich or in a salad. Improper drying procedures and using feverfew as a tea can greatly reduce the herb's beneficial properties. Capsules containing freeze-dried leaves are recommended.

Consumers are urged to be cautious when purchasing feverfew, as several studies have shown that you don't always get what you pay for. Several studies published in the *Journal of Natural Products* reported that the majority of American feverfew products tested contained either no parthenolide or less than 0.2 percent. Only buy feverfew from reputable companies that clearly state the percentage of parthenolide in the product (see Chapter 6).

How Does Feverfew Work?

The primary active ingredient in feverfew is parthenolide, a type of sesquiterpene lactone. Parthenolide and its components have anti-inflammatory capabilities that prevent the production of factors that promote inflammation (e.g., leukotrienes and thromboxanes) and inhibit the release of serotonin from blood platelets. They also inhibit aggregation of platelets, tone the blood vessels, and have a soothing effect on vascular smooth muscle. All of these features work together to prevent migraine.

Feverfew inhibits the activity of substances called amines. Amines increase in the brain during the initial stages of a migraine. One factor known to cause this increase is consumption of amine-containing foods, including coffee, some fried foods, and chocolate.

Here's the Proof
In 1772, about 200 years before it would undergo any type of scientific scrutiny, feverfew was valued by people who suffered with migraine pain. That was the year physician John Hill wrote in his book *The Family Herbal* that "[i]n the worst headache this herb exceeds whatever else is known."

Scientific study began in earnest in England in the 1980s. At the London Migraine Clinic, the first double-blind investigation was performed. The results of the six-month study showed significant improvement among patients who took feverfew compared with those who took a placebo. In a 1985 study published in the *British Medical Journal*, 70 percent of 270 patients with migraine who ate feverfew daily for an extended period of time had a substantial reduction in the frequency and/or severity of their attacks. Subsequent studies also clearly demonstrated that feverfew significantly reduces the severity and number of migraine attacks as well as the nausea and vomiting that often accompany these headaches.

Use of feverfew to reduce inflammation associated with rheumatoid arthritis was suggested by researchers who published their results in *Lancet* in 1985. They found that feverfew was more effective than nonsteroidal anti-inflammatories (NSAIDs) like aspirin in preventing the release of inflammatory substances. A placebo-controlled, double-blind study of feverfew for treatment of rheumatoid arthritis did not show any significant benefit—although experts who support its use note that the study used very low doses of feverfew, the parthenolide level was not established, and the patients continued to take NSAIDs at the same time, which may have had a negative effect on the herb's effectiveness. Positive results in animal studies, however, and anecdotal reports of its benefits in rheumatoid arthritis may prompt more investigation.

How Safe Is Feverfew?
Despite the widespread use of feverfew over the centuries, no toxic reactions have been reported. Some people experience mouth ulcers, swollen lips, and loss of taste when chewing the leaves. If you are pregnant, avoid feverfew because it stimulates the uterus. People who are allergic to chamomile, ragweed, or other plants in the daisy family should not take feverfew.

5-Hydroxytryptophan

What Is 5-Hydroxytryptophan?
The compound 5-hydroxytryptophan, better known as 5-HTP, is a derivative of the African plant *Griffonia simplicifolia*, which is native to Ghana and the Ivory

Coast. It is also a derivative of the amino acid tryptophan. The body produces 5-HTP from the tryptophan found in certain foods, including some cheeses, turkey, and almonds.

Because 5-HTP is closely related to tryptophan, it is under close scrutiny by the Food and Drug Administration. In 1989 the FDA banned the supplement form of tryptophan after a batch of the supplement was contaminated during processing and caused a fatal illness. Even though the tryptophan itself was not the cause of the fatalities, the ban has not been lifted. Thus far, many experts believe 5-HTP is safe. (See "How Safe is 5-HTP?")

What Types of Pain Does 5-HTP Help?
- Fibromyalgia
- Headache
- Migraine

How Do You Use 5-HTP?
For rapid absorption, take 5-HTP on an empty stomach. Adequate amounts of vitamin B_6, magnesium, and niacin are needed for 5-HTP to convert to serotonin. Between your diet and any supplements you may take, make sure you are getting the following recommended levels of these nutrients: vitamin B_6, 25 to 100 mg; magnesium, 250 to 500 mg; and niacin, 10 to 100 mg.

The general recommended dosage for 5-HTP is 50 to 100 mg, taken one to three times daily. If you have a child with chronic headache, consult with your physician for the correct dosage. Do not take 5-HTP for longer than three months unless you are under a doctor's supervision. Dosages for specific conditions are given below.

•**Fibromyalgia:** Take 50 to 100 mg 5-HTP three times daily, alone or combined with 150 to 250 mg chelated magnesium (preferably magnesium malate; otherwise take magnesium citrate, fumarate, succinate, or aspartate), and 300 mg St. John's wort extract (0.3 percent hypericin) three times daily. The combination of these three supplements is very effective in improving pain tolerance. Magnesium malate is recommended because the malic acid (malate) enhances the absorption of the magnesium. Both 5-HTP and St. John's wort raise serotonin levels and improve pain tolerance.

•**Migraine:** Take 100 to 200 mg three times daily as a preventive measure.

How Does 5-HTP Work?
5-HTP is effective in the treatment of pain at two levels. One, it raises the amount of serotonin in the body. Serotonin is a chemical neurotransmitter, produced by the body, which is found in very low levels in people who have migraine or fibromyalgia as well as those who suffer from depression. The body makes serotonin by first converting the amino acid L-tryptophan into 5-HTP and then converting the 5-HTP into serotonin. People who have low serotonin levels cannot take L-tryptophan supplements, because the supplement has been banned from sale except for very

limited prescription use. However, even if it were available, oral tryptophan has a very low conversion rate: Only 3 percent gets converted into serotonin compared with 70 percent of oral 5-HTP. This high conversion rate makes 5-HTP equally and sometimes more effective than conventional drugs prescribed to elevate serotonin levels, plus it has far fewer and less severe side effects than those associated with drug use. According to Ronald F. Bore, Ph.D., of the University of Mississippi, serotonin "is perhaps the most implicated in the etiology or treatment of various disorders, particularly those of the central nervous system."

Researchers also have found that 5-HTP increases the level of endorphins, the body's own pain-relieving substances. People who get migraines typically have low levels of endorphins. You may have heard about endorphins in reference to a "runner's high"; it has been found that runners and others who engage in vigorous physical activity for a length of time naturally raise their endorphin levels and thus have a high tolerance for pain. Thus the use of 5-HTP to increase endorphin levels is beneficial for pain relief.

Here's the Proof
Many clinical studies have been performed to evaluate the effectiveness of 5-HTP in the treatment of fibromyalgia. According to Professor Federigo Sicuteri, a leading expert on fibromyalgia, "5-HTP can largely improve the painful picture of primary fibromyalgia." In his study of 200 patients with fibromyalgia, he

found that 5-HTP improves pain tolerance when it is taken along with conventional antidepressants. The results of the combined treatment plan (conventional plus complementary medicine) were better than use of 5-HTP alone or conventional drugs alone. In studies reported in the *Journal of Internal Medicine Research*, patients with fibromyalgia who received 5-HTP experienced significant improvement over those who received placebo. Results are very good after 30 days of treatment and excellent after 90 days.

Excellent results are also possible when combining 5-HTP with magnesium and St. John's wort, according to Michael Murray, N.D., author of *Encyclopedia of Natural Medicine* and several other books on natural medicine. He and other researchers find that this combination produces results that are superior to those achieved using either substance alone.

The use of 5-HTP in the treatment of migraine also has been established, as 5-HTP increases the levels of endorphins and serotonin. Studies have shown 5-HTP to be as effective as methysergide (Sansert), a drug commonly used to treat migraine, in preventing or relieving migraine pain. The significant difference between the two treatments, however, is that methysergide causes many, and often severe, side effects, while 5-HTP is well tolerated, plus has the advantage of improving mood. Similar results were obtained when 5-HTP was compared with two drugs that prevent migraine, pizotifen (Sandomigrin) and propranolol (Inderal): While it was as effective as the conventional drugs, 5-HTP did not have the significant side effects.

Another benefit of 5-HTP is that it is very effective in treating chronic headache in children. Studies reported in *Drugs Experimental Clinical Research* and *Cephalgia* demonstrate that this natural remedy relieves pain without the dangerous side effects associated with conventional drugs. If interested in using 5-HTP for your child, consult your physician about the recommended dosage.

How Safe Is 5-HTP?

Researchers note that 5-HTP has been well tolerated at dosages as high as 600 mg daily. Some people experience mild nausea, heartburn, a feeling of fullness in the abdomen, and flatulence. If you are taking any type of prescription or over-the-counter medication, talk with your doctor before taking 5-HTP or St. John's wort. Potentially serious side effects (e.g., anxiety, confusion) can occur if you take 5-HTP while taking: Prozac or any other antidepressant, cold remedies that contain ephedrine or pseudoephedrine, levodopa (Dopar), buspirone (BuSpar), or lithium (Eskalith). Excessive drowsiness can occur if you take 5-HTP and antihistamines, muscle relaxants (e.g., carisoprodol [Rela], cyclobenzaprine [Flexeril]), or narcotic pain relievers (e.g., codeine, hydrocodone). Also, do not take St. John's wort if you are taking any type of conventional antidepressant.

Ginger

What Is Ginger?

Ginger (*Zingiber officinale*) is a perennial herb that is native to southern Asia but is cultivated in the tropical areas of India, China, Nigeria, Haiti, and Jamaica. It is closely related to marjoram and turmeric, another pain-relieving herb. Jamaica, the world's largest producer of ginger, exports more than 2 million pounds of the herb every year. The dried rhizome is used to make the remedies.

The Chinese have used ginger for medicinal purposes since before the fourth century B.C. Records show it was used to treat diarrhea, nausea, cholera, hemorrhage, rheumatism, toothache, and stomach pain. It is still used to treat many of these conditions today. It is also a key ingredient in the world's oldest written healthcare system, Ayurveda, because of its ability to stimulate the body's various systems. The ancient Egyptians, Greeks, and Romans valued it for its medicinal powers, as did the people of medieval England, who used it to treat the plague.

Ginger is composed largely of starch (up to 50 percent), then protein (9 percent), various fats, volatile oils, and resins. The components credited with the herb's medicinal value, called gingerols, are present in small quantities but are potent. Gingerols are known as the "pungent principles" and are found in high concentrations in the resins. Two other known pain relievers, curcumin and capsaicin, are present in ginger, although in minute amounts.

What Types of Pain Does Ginger Help?
- Headache and migraine
- Muscle pain
- Osteoarthritis
- Rheumatoid arthritis

How Do You Use Ginger?
Ginger is available in many forms, including liquid extracts, tinctures, capsules, and tablets. The dry powdered root can be added to liquids or food. Regardless of which form you choose, buy those that are standardized for 20 percent gingerol and shogaol, a derivative of gingerol. The capsules and tablets should always be taken with 6 to 8 ounces water. Ginger is also available as an oil, fresh or dry powdered root, and in teabags.

Typical dosages for standardized capsules or tablets is 100 to 200 mg daily; for tincture, 10 to 20 drops in water three times daily; and for fresh powdered root, 1 to 2 g daily. The dry powdered root can be added to liquids or food. To make a decoction, simmer 1 to 2 teaspoon dry powdered root in 1 cup water for 5 to 10 minutes; take as needed. To make a fresh root decoction, simmer 1 teaspoon grated fresh root in 1 cup water for 15 minutes. Strain and take as needed. You can also use fresh ginger: Mix 8 to 10 g grated fresh ginger in your diet daily. (See the sidebar for recipe ideas.)

•**Migraine:** For prevention, the standard dosages noted above are usually sufficient. You can supplement that dosage with tasty candied ginger, which you can nibble on during the day, or add ginger to your diet in other ways. (See the sidebar for recipe ideas.) To treat active migraine, take 200 mg every two hours for up to six times daily.

•**Muscle Pain:** In addition to the dosages noted above, you can rub ginger oil on painful areas. Mix 2 to 3 drops ginger oil with ½ ounce almond or another neutral oil.

•**Rheumatoid Arthritis:** Dr. Michael Murray recommends 2 to 4 g dry powdered ginger daily. This is roughly equivalent to 20 g fresh ginger root, or about a ½-inch slice. (See the congee recipe in the sidebar.)

GINGER RECIPES

The Chinese have long used a type of rice soup called congee as a breakfast food and an easy-to-digest meal for people who are recovering from an illness. Although the amount of ginger in one serving of congee does not meet the daily recommended dosage, this dish is a tasty addition to your pain-relief program. The Chinese regard it as a comfort food. You may want to increase the amount of ginger in the recipe, according to your taste.

GINGER AND FENNEL CONGEE
1 tablespoon whole fennel seeds
1 ½-inch piece fresh ginger, thinly sliced

1 cup brown or white rice
Dash salt
8 cups water
Brown sugar or maple syrup to taste

Toast the fennel seeds in a dry skillet until they are aromatic (about 3 minutes). Keep shaking the pan to avoid burning them. Place them in a spice grinder and process until the seeds are broken. Combine the fennel, ginger, rice, salt, and water in a large pot. Bring to a boil, reduce the heat, and simmer until the mixture is thick, about 3½ to 4 hours. Serve hot with brown sugar or maple syrup if desired.

CANDIED GINGER

Now you can take your "medicine" with you in a sweet, tasty form. This is the quick version of the recipe.

2 cups water
1½ cups sugar
1 3½-inch piece fresh ginger, peeled and cut into paper-thin slices

Place the water and sugar in a saucepan. Cook over low heat until the sugar has dissolved. Cover and bring to a boil. Add the ginger and bring to a boil again. Reduce the heat and simmer for 35 to 55 minutes, until the ginger is translucent. Strain off the syrup (you can use it in the recipe below) and place the ginger slices on a cooling rack. When they are cool, roll each piece in additional sugar to prevent them from sticking together. Store in an airtight container, where they will keep for several weeks.

GINGER SNOW CONES

Take the ginger syrup from the candy recipe and mix it with enough water to yield 4 cups. Process ice cubes in an ice crusher or ice shaver. Pour the syrup over the crushed or shaved ice to make snow cones.

How Does Ginger Work?

The anti-inflammatory effect of ginger is credited to the gingerols, which inhibit the formation of prostaglandins, thromboxane, and leukotrienes, chemicals that cause inflammation. Shogaol, a gingerol derivative, has analgesic properties, similar to those provided by **capsaicin**. Shogaol inhibits the release of substance P, a major neurotransmitter responsible for sending pain signals from the periphery of the body to the brain.

Ginger also inhibits the activity of thromboxane A2, which in turn helps promote smooth blood flow. This is especially important in the prevention of migraine, in which constricted blood vessels play a key role in the pain.

Here's the Proof

Until recently, most of the research conducted with ginger has been to prove its ability to prevent nausea. Now interest in its pain-relieving properties for treating arthritis has sparked some investigation. Several clinical studies published in *Medical Hypotheses* report that patients with osteoarthritis, rheumatoid arthritis, and muscular discomfort experienced significant reductions in pain and swelling when taking ginger. In one of the studies, in which 56 patients participated, 75 percent of the 46 arthritis patients and 100 percent of the patients with muscular discomfort enjoyed these benefits. Positive results from smaller studies, centuries of anecdotal reports of ginger's ability to reduce arthritic pain, and the herb's safety have convinced many healthcare practitioners to recommend ginger to their patients who have arthritis.

How Safe Is Ginger?

When taken as directed, ginger is very safe. People who take more than 6 g dried powdered ginger on an empty stomach may experience gastrointestinal distress, and some people get temporary heartburn at lower doses. Chemotherapy patients should not take any amount of ginger on an empty stomach because it can cause stomach irritation. Long-term use of ginger during pregnancy is not recommended. If you have a history of gallstones, consult your physician before taking ginger.

Glucosamine Sulfate

What Is Glucosamine?
Glucosamine is a naturally occurring substance that
is found in the body's tissues. It is also found in chitin, the horny substance that makes up the external
skeleton of beetles, crabs, and several marine inver-
tebrates. In the human body, its primary function is
to provide the joints with the material necessary to
produce glycosaminoglycan, a critical ingredient in
cartilage. It also helps in the formation of tendons,
skin, bones, nails, and ligaments. The supplement glucosamine sulfate is the artificially produced version
of this natural substance. Both the natural and synthetic supplements provide comparable results.

Another substance often marketed with glucosamine and touted as an effective treatment for arthritis
is chondroitin sulfate. It is also produced by the body
and is a significant component of cartilage, where it
provides structure, allows nutrients and other molecules to pass through, and retains essential elements
and water. Use of chondroitin for arthritis is contro-
versial, however, given that its absorption rate by the
body is only 13 percent or less, compared with 90
percent or better for glucosamine. While some physicians believe that chondroitin works best when combined with glucosamine sulfate, this theory has not
been proven yet.

What Types of Pain Does Glucosamine Help?
- Bursitis
- Osteoarthritis
- Tendonitis

How Do You Use Glucosamine?
Glucosamine sulfate is sold in capsules or as a flavored powder that you can add to water. The standard dose is one 500-mg capsule three times daily, or 1,500 mg daily. Most products are synthetically produced, but some manufacturers market supplements extracted from chitin. Take the supplement with food, which will help prevent the occasional gastrointestinal disturbances associated with this remedy. (See "Is Glucosamine Safe?") If you choose to take chondroitin with glucosamine, the recommendation is to base dosage on body weight, at a ratio of 5:4 glucosamine: chondroitin. For example, if you weigh less than 120 pounds, take 1,000 mg glucosamine and 800 mg chondroitin; 120 to 200 pounds, 1,500 mg glucosamine and 1,200 mg chondroitin; and more than 200 pounds, 2,000 mg glucosamine and 1,600 mg chondroitin.

How Does It Work?
Studies indicate that glucosamine relieves the pain and stiffness associated with **osteoarthritis** by stimulating the cells that produce glycosaminoglycans (GAGs), which are the components of cartilage that allow the joints to move smoothly. Osteoarthritis involves the

degeneration of GAGs; thus proponents of glucosamine theorize that a high intake of the supplement will stimulate production of GAGs and result in cartilage regeneration. Glucosamine also stimulates production of proteoglycans, another substance important in building cartilage. (See listing in the Bibliography for *The Arthritis Cure* by Jason Theodosakis.)

Another way glucosamine relieves pain is through its anti-inflammatory activity. This property may make it a safe and effective alternative to aspirin and other NSAIDs and their side effects, which include gastrointestinal distress and bleeding of the stomach lining.

Here's the Proof

Since the early 1980s, clinical trials have been conducted to determine the effectiveness of glucosamine in relieving osteoarthritis. Studies of both oral and injectable glucosamine have shown that it is superior to placebo in reducing pain and tenderness and in increasing mobility. Comparisons of glucosamine and the NSAID ibuprofen have revealed that this natural remedy is as effective as ibuprofen and is far less likely to cause side effects. In one controlled study, for example, 37 percent of patients taking ibuprofen had adverse effects while only 7 percent of those taking glucosamine experienced any side effects. In a study published in *Clinical Therapeutics*, researchers found that patients taking glucosamine not only had improved symptoms but also had healthy cartilage.

Patients taking placebo had cartilage that revealed osteoarthritis.

How Safe Is Glucosamine?

Occasionally, glucosamine can cause minor side effects, including heartburn, diarrhea, nausea, indigestion, and stomach upset. If you have high blood pressure, check the label to see if the glucosamine formulation contains sodium.

Hypericum (St. John's Wort)

What Is Hypericum (St. John's Wort)?

Hypericum (*Hypericum perforatum*) is one of many herbs that lead a double life: both as an herbal remedy (St. John's wort) and as a homeopathic remedy (hypericum). The homeopathic remedy is discussed here. See the separate entry for **St. John's wort**.

The homeopathic remedy is made from St. John's wort, a shrubby perennial plant with yellow flowers. It is cultivated around the world and grows naturally in Europe, Asia, and the United States. The plant was named for John the Baptist because the flowers bloom around the saint's birthday, June 24, which is a traditional time to harvest it.

What Types of Pain Does Hypericum Help?

Hypericum is used for individuals who experience nerve-related pain, including

- Back pain, specifically tailbone pain (coccydynia)
- Burns
- Hemorrhoids
- Neuralgia
- Postsurgical (including dental surgery)
- Trauma, especially injuries to areas of the body that are rich in nerve endings, such as the spine, fingers, and toes

Matching Characteristics
Because hypericum is used primarily as a first-aid remedy, there is no specific hypericum personality profile. Physical conditions that respond to hypericum include neuralgia; toothache with tearing or pulling pain; back pain that travels up and down the spine; puncture wounds; nerve pains in the rectum; painful, bleeding hemorrhoids; and head pain in which the head feels elongated. Mental symptoms that may be alleviated include drowsiness and depression. Symptoms improve when the head is tilted back and worsen in cold, damp, or foggy conditions and in warm, stuffy rooms.

How Do You Use Hypericum?
The homeopathic remedy can be taken according to the Rule of Three (see page 220) or you can refer to the following alternative doses and conditions:

•**Back Pain (Coccydynia, the Tailbone):** Hypericum is specifically indicated for aching or shooting pains of the coccyx caused by a fall or injury to the tailbone. Take 6c three times daily for up to seven days.

•**Burns.** For first- and second-degree burns, add 10 drops tincture to ½ cup sterile cool water and apply to the affected area as a compress or with cotton balls.

•**Neuralgia (General Nerve Pain):** When you have pain that is sharp, shooting, and burning, try 6c hypericum once every hour for up to four doses. For less severe pain, try the herbal remedy.

•**Postsurgical (Including Dental Surgery):** When experiencing shooting pains, take 30c two to three times daily after you have completed a course of treatment with **arnica**.

•**Trauma (Falls, Blows, and Bruises) to Nerve-rich Areas (e.g., Fingers and Toes):** Treat with 30c twice daily for two or three days after completing a course of **arnica**.

How Does Hypericum Work?
See the explanation on page 61.

Here's the Proof
See the explanation on page 61.

How Safe Is Hypericum?
See the explanation on page 64.

Magnesium

What Is Magnesium?
Magnesium is an essential and often underappreciated mineral. Although the average person's body contains

only about one ounce of magnesium, this minute amount is responsible for enhancing the activity of approximately 300 enzyme processes and for preventing and fighting many chronic conditions. It is involved in energy production, muscle relaxation, tooth and bone formation, and nerve functioning. It works closely with potassium and calcium to regulate heart rhythm and clot the blood.

Magnesium is found in many foods, including whole grains, legumes, dark green leafy vegetables, nuts, and shellfish. Many people, however, fail to get enough magnesium in their diet and have an inadequate store of the mineral in their body. Stress, use of certain medications (i.e., laxatives and potassium-depleting diuretics), and vigorous physical activity also can cause the body to lose magnesium and result in a deficiency.

What Types of Pain Does Magnesium Help?
- Cluster headache
- Dysmenorrhea
- Fibromyalgia
- Migraine
- Muscle pain
- (PMS) Premenstrual syndrome

Magnesium's ability to relax muscles makes it useful in relieving the chronic pain of fibromyalgia, menstrual cramps, and various sports injuries. Its effectiveness in the treatment of migraine is still under investigation, but there is evidence that it may complement and enhance the effect of the prescription migraine drug sumatriptan (Imitrex).

How Do You Use Magnesium?

The recommended optimal daily intake of magnesium is 250 to 500 mg. According to Dr. Michael Murray, many nutritional experts recommend basing magnesium intake on body weight: 6 mg for every 2.2 pounds. A 110-pound person would need 300 mg, for example, while a 154-pound person would need 420 mg. Dosages for specific conditions are noted below.

•**Cluster Headache and Migraine:** As a preventive measure, take 250 to 400 mg three times daily.

•**Fibromyalgia:** Take 150 mg magnesium with 600 mg malic acid twice daily. (The malic acid enhances the absorption of the magnesium.)

•**PMS:** Take 12 mg per 2.2 pounds body weight; that is, 600 mg for a 110-pound person; 840 mg for a 154-pound person.

When taking magnesium supplements (which come in capsule, tablet, and powder forms), be sure to take adequate amounts of calcium as well, because these two minerals work synergistically. The proper ratio is 2:1 calcium:magnesium—for example, 1,000 mg calcium and 500 mg magnesium. An improper balance can minimize the benefits you can get from both supplements. Consider buying a supplement that has both minerals in the proper amounts.

Magnesium also works closely with another nutrient, vitamin B$_6$, which is necessary so that magnesium can enter cells. Take 50 to 100 mg daily, either in a multivitamin-mineral or B-complex supplement. If you take more than 50 mg daily, divide the dose and take twice daily for up to 100 mg total.

Magnesium comes in several forms, including magnesium aspartate, magnesium carbonate, magnesium citrate, magnesium gluconate, magnesium oxide, and magnesium sulfate. The citrate type is the most easily absorbed by the body; the oxide is the most poorly absorbed. All are better absorbed when taken with food.

How Does Magnesium Work?

For people who suffer with migraine or cluster headache, magnesium relaxes constricted blood vessels and brings relief. Both types of head pain are associated with low magnesium levels in the bloodstream.

Women who experience PMS have magnesium levels that are significantly lower than women without PMS. Because magnesium plays a major role in maintaining normal cell function, these low levels are believed to be a factor in the many symptoms associated with PMS.

Here's the Proof

Low levels of magnesium are characterized by general aches and pains as well as a lower premenstrual pain threshold. These and other PMS symptoms are improved dramatically with magnesium supplementation (along with the proper ratio of calcium), as shown in several clinical trials. Studies published in the *Journal of Reproductive Medicine* and the *Journal of the American College of Nutrition* suggest that combining vitamin B_6 with magnesium yields even greater relief. (See "How Do You Use Magnesium?" above.)

How Safe Is Magnesium?
According to the *USP Guide to Vitamins and Minerals*, you should consult your doctor before taking magnesium supplements if you are already taking any of the following:

•**Cellulose sodium phosphate (CSP):** Magnesium may interfere with CSP: take magnesium at least 1 hour before or after CSP.

•**Other magnesium-containing preparations, including enemas:** Use of both may cause high levels of magnesium in the blood and increase the chance of side effects.

•**Sodium polystyrene sulfonate (SPS):** Magnesium may not be as effective if you are also taking SPS.

•**Tetracycline (oral).** Magnesium may prevent tetracycline from working properly, so take magnesium one to three hours before or after an oral dose of tetracycline.

•**If you have heart disease**, magnesium may make the condition worse.

•**If you have kidney problems**, magnesium may increase the risk of hypermagnesemia (high levels of magnesium).

Side effects associated with magnesium supplements are very rare and generally occur in people who take the mineral by injection. Symptoms of overdose are rare in people who have normal kidney function; these symptoms include blurred or double vision, coma, dizziness or fainting, severe drowsiness, increased or decreased urination, slow heartbeat, and trouble breathing.

Marijuana

What Is Marijuana?

Marijuana (*Cannabis sativa*) is a branching plant with tiny green flowers and long leaflets. It is cultivated around the world for its fiber (hemp) as well as for its leaves, which are used as a legal and an illegal drug, depending on where it is being used and for what purpose. More than 100 species of *Cannabis* grow wild throughout North America.

The medicinal use of marijuana dates back to ancient Egypt and China, when healers used the leaves and seeds to relieve pain, nervousness, fever, obesity, asthma, dandruff, hemorrhoids, inflammation, and leprosy. In the third century, a marijuana "tea" was drunk by people who were about to undergo surgery, while many gentlewomen in the nineteenth century routinely took marijuana to relieve menstrual cramps.

Today, use of marijuana as a drug is illegal in many parts of the world. Efforts to make its medicinal use legal in the United States have been under way for years. To date, seven states (Alaska, Arizona, California, Colorado, Nevada, Oregon, and Washington) have passed laws making it legal to prescribe marijuana for certain medical conditions. These laws, however, have been challenged and as of this writing are still being hotly debated. Although certain states have voted marijuana's use to be legal, it is still illegal everywhere in the United States as long as the federal laws prohibiting its use remain in force.

What Types of Pain Does Marijuana Help?
- Dysmenorrhea
- Glaucoma
- Migraine
- Muscle pain (especially muscles spasms in patients with multiple sclerosis and amputees)
- Osteoarthritis
- Rheumatoid arthritis

There are many anecdotal reports of people getting significant relief from other types of pain, including back pain, carpal tunnel syndrome, fibromyalgia, and nerve pain. So far, however, the FDA has not approved use of the legal form of marijuana, Marinol (see "How Do You Use Marijuana?"), in patients with pain. Proof that marijuana is effective for other types of pain may be coming, however, now that the ban on private research has been lifted. (See "Here's the Proof.")

How Do You Use Marijuana?
Marijuana can be smoked, added to food, or taken as THC (9-tetrahydrocannabinol) capsules. THC is the

main active ingredient in marijuana. The THC capsules, marketed under the brand name Marinol, are the legal form of the drug, given by prescription. Many patients who have used THC complain that it takes too long for the drug to take effect (one hour or more), which makes it easy to overdose on the drug while waiting for relief. Many also object to "getting high," which often happens with Marinol because the dosage is not easy to regulate. Many patients prefer to smoke marijuana because the THC enters their system much faster, and they can control the amount of drug they receive. Once they begin to get relief, they can stop smoking, before they get high. Most people who use marijuana for medical purposes want enough pain relief so they can go on with their lives as normally as possible; they are not seeking a way to get high legally, as some opponents of medical marijuana claim.

How Does Marijuana Work?

Marijuana is a complex plant, containing more than 400 compounds and 60 kinds of cannabinoids (the organic substances researchers believe are responsible for its pharmacologic actions). The main cannabinoid in marijuana is 9-tetrahydrocannabinol, or THC. This substance is the one primarily responsible for marijuana's mind-altering effects, but it also appears to be responsible for the plant's ability to relieve various types of pain and to treat intractable nausea caused by chemotherapy and radiation therapy.

Medical researchers do not fully understand marijuana's ability to relieve pain. They have found, however, that the cannabinoids in marijuana are very similar to a chemical in the body called anandamide. This chemical triggers nerve receptors in the brain and body that are responsible for pain, nausea and vomiting, internal eye pressure, and motor functioning. This critical relationship deserves further research, especially because it seems to work differently from pain relievers such as NSAIDs and opiates.

For now, researchers note that marijuana seems to work best on nerve pain. This is a significant problem among people with paraplegia and quadriplegia, for whom marijuana can relieve their painful muscle spasms and neurological pain. According to Bill Zimmerman, Ph.D., Rick Bayer, M.D., and Nancy Crumpacker, M.D., in *Is Marijuana the Right Medicine for You?*, thousands of paralyzed war veterans in Veterans Administration hospitals across the United States commonly use marijuana; it is the only way they can control the spasms and not experience the debilitating side effects and the possibility of addiction associated with conventional drugs. Because of the legal ramifications of marijuana use in most states, health professionals who witness patients using the drug, and note the relief they get, generally turn a blind eye to the situation.

In glaucoma, fluid builds up in the eye, creating painful pressure and damage to the retina and the optic nerve. Marijuana appears to reduce the pressure by constricting the capillaries in the eye, reducing the amount of fluid, and allowing it to drain from the eye. This may explain why people who smoke marijuana often have red eyes.

Here's the Proof

One of the hurdles some scientists bring up about research into marijuana is that placebo-controlled trials are not possible because no placebo can match marijuana's psychoactive effects. Proponents of medicinal marijuana argue that the vast amount of anecdotal evidence, coupled with the studies that have been conducted and the centuries of use, are more than enough to allow the legal use of marijuana for people in pain.

Thus, scientific research into the medicinal benefits of marijuana has been sporadic and been undertaken under the watchful eye of the federal government, which has had a hard time justifying research on a drug that is part of its "war on drugs" program. In 1970 Congress banned marijuana for medicinal use under the Controlled Substances Act. Soon after passage of the ban, a University of California researcher discovered that marijuana could help people with glaucoma by reducing the intraocular pressure characteristic of the disease. Then in 1976 a glaucoma patient in Washington, D.C., was arrested for growing and using marijuana for his disease. He won his case in court on a "medical necessity" defense, and the federal government allowed him to continue growing marijuana for his own use. From that time until 1992, the government continued to approve a selected number of patients, most of whom had AIDS, for a program in which they received medicinal marijuana, free of charge. Although the program was discontinued in 1992, up to 34 patients were receiving the drug from the government each month. Several of these people are alive today and still receive it.

In the late 1970s and 1980s several states, with the approval of the FDA, conducted research studies into the use of marijuana to control the nausea and vomiting associated with chemotherapy. The results were highly impressive, which prompted the FDA to approve Marinol in 1986. This approval, however, was only for people who experienced nausea associated with cancer treatment.

Research into the medicinal value of marijuana slowed to a near standstill until early 1997, when the National Institutes of Health issued a recommendation for an exploration into the drug's benefits. On March 17, 1999, the National Academy of Sciences' Institute of Medicine issued a report on the pros and cons of medicinal use of marijuana. The investigative panel spent 18 months reviewing all the scientific research and studies available and listening to the testimony of patients and physicians who use and prescribe the drug. The panel concluded that marijuana appears to be helpful in the treatment of pain, nausea, painful muscle spasms associated with diseases such as multiple sclerosis, and weight loss related to AIDS. One of the report's principle investigators, Dr. John Benson, a professor emeritus at the Oregon Health Sciences University School of Medicine, said that their research showed "there's just too much promise there to ignore it."

This is not news to the few who use marijuana legally and the tens of thousands who use it illegally to relieve chronic, severe pain and various serious disorders as well as those who take the FDA-approved Marinol. Although many patients with glaucoma, migraines, and other diseases use marijuana and report much success with it, the institute report did not support use of marijuana for these conditions. It argues, for example, that glaucoma patients receive only short-term benefits from marijuana, which are outweighed by the long-term hazards. (See "How Safe Is Marijuana?") The institute recommended that clinical trials of marijuana be conducted and that scientists should work on developing fast-acting and effective ways to administer the drug without smoking it.

That recommendation was heeded by the Clinton administration. On May 21, 1999, the hold on research-quality marijuana was lifted. For more than 20 years before that time, what little marijuana research being done was restricted under federal laws and international agreements and was open only to federally funded researchers. With the ban lifted, physicians and private researchers can purchase and study marijuana.

How Safe Is Marijuana?

As a mind-altering drug, marijuana can trigger a variety of reactions, some pleasant and others not so pleasant. Advocates of smoking marijuana for medicinal purposes emphasize that smoking marijuana rather than taking THC pills allows patients to stop ingesting the drug before it makes them high. Many patients have complained that THC makes them feel too high and they are unable to perform their usual activities. Both THC and smoking too much marijuana can cause panic attacks, hallucinations, dry mouth, nausea, and vomiting. Motor coordination and judgment are often impaired, which makes operating a motor vehicle or equipment dangerous.

Smoking any amount of marijuana can cause damage to the lungs and increase the risk of lung cancer, emphysema, and constrictive lung disease. Long-term use appears to cause menstrual difficulties, and animal studies suggest that it may cause birth defects in humans.

MSM

What Is MSM?

Methylsulfonylmethane, or MSM, is an organic form of the mineral sulfur, which the body needs to perform certain essential functions. Although the word "sulfur" sounds like several other compounds (e.g., sulfa drugs and sulfites), it is in no way related to them and is safe for those who cannot take the other substances.

All life, including plants, animals, and algae, contains sulfur. MSM is one of three kinds of sulfur compounds that make up 85 percent of the sulfur in all living things; DMSO (dimethylsufoxide) and DMS (dimethylsufide) are the other two. MSM is found in high concentrations in some food plants, including broccoli, onions, garlic, and cabbage.

Most people are deficient in sulfur. One reason is that MSM has a fragile structure that is easily destroyed during food processing and cooking. Another reason is that much of the soil used to grow crops is nutritionally deficient. The only people who have a good chance of getting enough sulfur in their food are those whose diet consists mostly of raw, organic foods.

What Types of Pain Does MSM Help?
- Back pain
- Bursitis
- Carpal tunnel syndrome
- Cystitis
- Fibromyalgia
- Headache
- Muscle pain
- Osteoarthritis
- Tendinitis

How Do You Use MSM?
MSM is available in oral form as capsules or crystals and for topical use as a lotion, cream, or gel. Capsules are convenient if you are taking 2 or 3 g daily, but crystals may be easier if you are taking higher doses. The crystals can be mixed into water, juice, or any nonalcoholic beverage.

The general dosage is 2,000 to 8,000 mg daily, depending on how much pain you have and how well your stomach tolerates the supplement. Stanley Jacob, M.D., who studied DMSO and MSM for more than 30 years and recently wrote a book on the subject, *The Miracle of MSM: The Natural Solution for Pain*, recommends starting low and slow, beginning with 2,000 mg daily and adding another 1,000 mg every few days until you reach your desired level. If you start to develop more frequent stools or minor stomach upset, cut back the dosage. To help avoid stomach distress, take MSM with or immediately after meals. For even better results, take oral MSM and apply the cream or gel to painful areas.

How Does MSM Work?

According to Dr. Jacob, MSM relieves pain, inflammation, muscle soreness, and cramps in several different ways. One way is that it appears to inhibit the pain signals as they travel from the site of the damaged tissue to the brain. It also reduces the incidence of muscle contractions or spasms, which often are a component of pain. Yet a third way is that MSM promotes blood flow, which speeds up the healing process.

MSM also has the ability to affect the flow of substances, both beneficial and harmful, in and out of the body's cells. This ability to increase and sustain cell permeability and flexibility allows harmful factors such as toxins and lactic acid to flow out of the cells and also allows needed nutrients to flow in. A healthy exchange of materials and fluids through the cell membrane prevents the buildup of pressure inside and outside the cells, which in turn reduces the chance of inflammation in the surrounding tissues and nerves, and thus reduces or eliminates pain. It also helps eliminate the buildup of toxins in and around the joints, which is a key factor in arthritis and bursitis.

Here's the Proof

Most of the research on MSM has been done by the "fathers" of MSM—Robert J. Herschler and Stanley Jacob, M.D., who began their studies more than 30 years ago with DMSO. Dr. Jacob began experimenting with DMSO in the 1950s while at the University of Oregon Medical School. There he teamed up with Robert Herschler, a chemist who was working with DMSO at a paper-making company. By 1965 they had conducted more than 1,500 studies involving approximately 100,000 patients, most of whom had arthritis or another inflammatory condition. Despite the very high response rate from these patients, the FDA did not approve DMSO, largely because there was a thalidomide scare going on at the time and the agency was reluctant to approve any new substances. (Thalidomide is a sedative that was found to cause serious birth defects if taken during pregnancy.) In the United States, DMSO has been approved by the FDA for only one condition—the painful inflammatory disease of the bladder called interstitial cystitis. Yet it continues to be used widely around the world for the treatment of arthritis, fibromyalgia, and various other muscular and skeletal disorders.

While DMSO is effective, it also has the annoying side effect of causing a strong fish odor and taste in those who take it. In the late 1970s, Herschler and Dr. Jacob began to investigate MSM and found that it had most of the benefits of DMSO and no odor. Since then Dr. Jacob has used MSM in his clinic, as have thousands of other doctors who regularly recommend it to their patients. According to Jacob, much of the "scientific fine print" relating to MSM's ability to heal needs to be established. Yet clinical experience and scores of testimonials from physicians and patients attest to the fact that it relieves pain and inflammation for the majority of people who take it, especially that related to arthritis.

How Safe Is MSM?

No significant side effects have been reported by people who have used MSM. Because it is a water-soluble micronutrient, excess MSM can be eliminated easily from the body. Researchers believe MSM may act like vitamin C: that is, the more your body needs it, the greater tolerance your body will have for it. If you take more than the body needs and utilizes, you will experience one or more temporary reactions. With vitamin C, taking too high a dosage results in diarrhea. Physicians call this reaction *bowel tolerance*. A similar reaction can occur with MSM if your dosage is too high; minor rash and temporary headache are other possible symptoms. All of these reactions typically disappear when you reduce the dosage.

MSM has not been found to interfere with any over-the-counter or prescription medications. As a precautionary measure, anyone taking high doses of aspirin or any blood-thinning medication should consult their physician before taking MSM. Although there are no clinical indications that MSM is contraindicated during pregnancy, it is always best to consult with your physician before taking MSM, especially if you are pregnant.

Rhus Toxicodendron

What Is Rhus Toxicodendron?
Rhus toxicodendron is a homeopathic remedy that is derived from poison ivy, and it grows throughout North America. Medicinal use of rhus toxicodendron is believed to have begun in 1798, when a French doctor discovered that the herpetic eruptions of one of his patients were cured by poisoning with the plant. For many decades following his discovery, rhus toxicodendron was used by homeopathic and some conventional doctors to treat scarlet fever, skin diseases, and rheumatism, but it eventually was discarded by the conventional medical community.

What Types of Pain Does Rhus Toxicodendron Help?
- Backache (with stiffness along the spine)

- Bursitis and tendonitis
- Carpal tunnel syndrome
- Gout
- Headache
- Muscle pain
- Osteoarthritis
- Rheumatoid arthritis
- Sciatica
- Shingles
- Tendinitis

Matching Characteristics

People who respond best to rhus toxicodendron may have the following symptoms: dizziness that feels as if the brain were loose in the head, numbness; weakness in the limbs; restlessness; aching pains; sore head muscles; eczema of the face; rheumatic headache triggered by exposure to cold damp weather; inflamed eyes; painful eyeballs; stiff neck; swollen glands in the neck; dry mouth and throat; extreme thirst; painful swallowing; dry cough; sensitive scalp; and cravings for cold milk and sweets.

Mental or emotional symptoms that respond to rhus toxicodendron include anxiety, fear, crying for no apparent reason, irritability, incoherent speech, and depression or thoughts of suicide. Symptoms are worse at night, during rest, when lying on your back or right side, or when the weather is cold, wet, and rainy. Symptoms improve when the weather is warm and dry and when moving the affected body parts.

How Do You Use Rhus Toxicodendron?
Rhus toxicodendron remedies are available in liquid, granule, powder, and tablet forms. Tablets are the most common form, but any one is equally effective when taken according to the Rule of Three. (See page 220.) If taking a tablet, place it under the tongue and allow it to dissolve. See Chapter 6 for dosing instructions for children. Alternative dosages for several specific conditions follow.

•**Back Pain/Spasm (Acute):** Rhus toxicodendron is indicated when the pain is aching or tearing; the back is very stiff but improves as you move around; the pain is better when heat is applied or when lying on a hard surface but worse at night. Take 30c immediately when the pain begins, then every four to six hours, for up to four doses. If you do not notice any significant improvement by the fourth dose, try another remedy, such as **bryonia**. Once improvement begins, reduce the dosage to once or twice a day for up to two more days. An alternative approach is to take 6c four times daily for up to 10 days.

•**Bursitis:** Try rhus toxicodendron when bursitis is accompanied by tearing pain and stiff, swollen joints made worse by rest and cold damp weather. Take 6c four times daily for up to seven days.

•**Carpal Tunnel Syndrome:** Indicated when the pain is relieved by heat and made worse by cold, damp weather. Moving the wrist in a circular pattern may cause the wrist joint to crack. Take 6c rhus toxicodendron three to four times daily for up to seven days.

•**Gout:** Helpful when the joints are painful, swollen, and hot. The pain improves with warmth and when moving around and grows worse when lying down or resting. Take 6c every hour for up to six doses in acute cases. For chronic cases, take 6c three to four times daily until there is significant improvement.

•**Muscle Pain (Sprains and Strains):** After completing a course of **arnica**, take 6c or 12c rhus toxicodendron two to three times daily until the injury improves.

•**Osteoarthritis:** This remedy is effective for flareups only, not chronic cases, and when there is stiffness in the morning. If the pain is relieved by heat but aggravated by cold and damp and while resting, but improves with continued movement, rhus toxicodendron is indicated. Take 6c four times a day for up to two weeks.

•**Rheumatoid Arthritis:** People likely to respond are most stiff when they first try to move but experience less pain with slow, continued movement. Other characteristics include restlessness and difficulty getting comfortable when sitting. Take 30c three times daily for two weeks.

•**Sciatica:** Symptoms include numbness and tingling in the leg(s), which gets worse when the person is exposed to cold. Tearing pain is relieved by heat and movement but aggravated by inactivity and cold and damp. Take 6c every hour for up to 10 doses or every 30 minutes until you get improvement if the pain is acute.

•**Shingles:** Indicated when skin eruptions are numerous and fluid-filled, painful, and extremely itchy; when the symptoms are worse at night; and when symptoms improve with warm applications and movement. If you have shingles, take 30c twice daily for two to three days. If you take the 6c potency, take three to four times daily. Discontinue the remedy if you have improvement or if the lesions become much worse.

•**Tendinitis:** Indicated when there is tearing pain aggravated by damp weather, rest, or movement and when the pain wears off with continued movement. Take 6c four times a day for up to seven days.

Here's the Proof
See the explanation on page 61.

How Safe Is Rhus Toxicodendron?
See the explanation on page 64.

St. John's Wort

What Is St. John's wort?
St. John's wort (*Hypericum perforatum*) is one of many herbs that lead a double life: as an herbal remedy (St. John's wort) and as a homeopathic one (hypericum). Its medicinal uses as an herbal remedy differ somewhat from those when taken as a home-

opathic remedy. See the separate entry for **hypericum**.

St. John's wort ("wort" is an Old English word that means "plant") is believed to have been named after John the Baptist, because the plant's flowers typically bloom on or near his birthday, June 24. From ancient times through the Middle Ages, the leaves and flowers of St. John's wort were taken internally to treat depression, insomnia, diarrhea, stomach disorders, kidney and bladder problems, and anxiety. The bright yellow flowers of this shrubby perennial release a bright red extract when chopped, and this fluid was used topically to treat wounds and to fight infection and inflammation.

St. John's wort is perhaps best known as an herbal treatment for mild depression. Its ability to reduce pain, either alone or in combination with **5-HTP** and **magnesium**, has received increased attention.

What Types of Pain Does St. John's wort Help?
- Burns
- Dysmenorrhea
- Ear infections
- Fibromyalgia
- Hemorrhoids
- Migraine
- Trauma

How Do You Use St. John's wort?
The herbal remedy St. John's wort is available in tablet, capsule, softgel, tincture, cream, and oil forms.

Look for a form that contains an extract standardized for 0.3 percent hypericin, the (believed to be) active ingredient in St. John's wort. The recommended dose for St. John's wort is 300 mg in tablets or capsules three times daily, or 450 mg twice daily of a standardized extract. To make an infusion, steep 2 teaspoons St. John's wort in 8 ounces boiling water for 10 minutes. Drink three cups daily. St. John's wort should be taken either with food or immediately after eating to avoid stomach upset.

For ear pain, use St. John's wort oil. It acts as an anti-inflammatory, soothes the nerves of the ear canal, and stops the pain. St. John's wort oil should be mixed with another oil, such as mullein flower oil, in equal amounts. Place three drops of the mixture into the affected ear and cover the ear with a cotton ball. Reapply every six to eight hours as necessary.

In Germany, where much of the research on St. John's wort has been done, health experts often use St. John's wort oil as a topical treatment for first-degree burns, hemorrhoids, and muscle pain. Throughout Europe, St. John's wort oil is used to treat inflammation and abrasions. To use St. John's wort for these purposes, buy a commercial cream standardized for 0.3 percent hypericin, or mix equal amounts of St. John's wort oil with a carrier oil, such as mullein oil, and apply it to the affected areas.

To treat sunburn, make a compress soaked in 1 part St. John's wort tincture or extract to 9 parts cool water. Lay the compress on the affected area for at least 15 minutes. St. John's wort helps relieve the pain caused by nerve damage and swelling caused by over-exposure to the sun.

How Does St. John's wort Work?

St. John's wort's ability to alleviate pain is attributed to the fact that it raises serotonin levels in the body. Low levels of serotonin are associated with chronic headache, migraine, and fibromyalgia. In fact, several of the conventional drugs used to treat and prevent migraine are designed to raise serotonin levels. St. John's wort also has anti-inflammatory and antimicrobial activity (attributed to its volatile oils and tannin), and one study has shown that it helps heal burns when applied to the skin.

Here's the Proof

Michael Murray, N.D., author of *The Healing Power of Herbs*, reports that more than 35 years of research shows that low serotonin levels cause a lowered pain threshold in patients with chronic headache. Based on these findings, researchers and pharmaceutical companies have developed prescription drugs that raise serotonin levels in an effort to treat and help prevent migraine. St. John's wort offers the same results without the side effects associated with migraine medications. Dr. Murray and other researchers have found that combining St. John's wort with **5-HTP** and **magnesium** is an effective remedy for relief of the pain associated with fibromyalgia.

Results of research studies support the use of St. John's wort oil and cream for the topical treatment of burns, muscle pain, and skin injuries. According to Lisa Murray-Doran, N.D., a naturopath and an instructor at the Canadian College of Naturopathic Medicine in Toronto, an infused oil of St. John's wort eases the pain of scrapes and abrasions and can heal second-degree burns three times faster than conventional treatments. To make your own St. John's wort oil, see the sidebar. Or you can buy the oil and apply it as noted in the sidebar.

ST. JOHN'S WORT OIL

To make your own St. John's wort oil for use on burns, cuts, and abrasions, place 1 cup fresh yellow flowers from the plant into a quart jar and cover with olive oil. Close the lid tightly and set the jar in a sunny window or other warm place. Shake it daily for two to three weeks. The oil will turn red. Strain out the flowers and store the oil in a cool, dark place in a jar with a tight lid. When treating burns, cool down the area first with cold water, pat it dry, and then gently apply the oil with a cotton ball or soft cloth. For cuts and abrasions, apply the oil directly to the wound with a cotton ball.

Is St. John's wort Safe?

St. John's wort rarely causes side effects; when it does they can include dizziness, constipation, upset stomach, fatigue, and dry mouth. If you are taking conventional antidepressant medication, talk with your doctor before you begin to take St. John's wort, because combining them can cause adverse reactions. People often experience increased sensitivity to the sun when taking St. John's wort and so should avoid exposure to the sun while under treatment.

Turmeric

What Is Turmeric?

Turmeric (*Curcuma longa*) is a perennial herb that is widely cultivated in China, Indonesia, India, and other tropical regions. The plant is a member of the ginger family and, like its cousin, has a thick rhizome, which is used for its medicinal properties. Turmeric contains a volatile oil called curcumin, a pungent orange-yellow substance that is one of the herb's most active ingredients.

Turmeric is highly regarded in the traditional Ayurvedic medicine system for a wide variety of ailments. In India turmeric is used as a tonic for the entire body. Among practitioners of traditional Chinese medicine, turmeric is prescribed for colic and liver disorders. As a spice, it is enjoyed around the world, but especially in Indian foods, as a key ingredient in curry powder and in mustards.

What Types of Pain Does Turmeric Help?
- Carpal tunnel syndrome
- Dysmenorrhea
- Irritable bowel syndrome

- Liver disorders
- Rheumatoid arthritis

How Do You Use Turmeric?

As a pain relief remedy, turmeric can be used as a seasoning or its active ingredient, curcumin, can be taken as a supplement. Turmeric is available in powdered root or liquid extract or in capsule form. Look for standardized forms with up to 90 percent curcumin. Typical dosages are 250 to 500 mg standardized capsules taken up to three times daily; 10 to 30 drops extract up to three times daily; or up to three cups of the decoction daily. To prepare the decoction from the powdered root, steep 1 teaspoon in 8 ounces milk (warm, not boiled) for 15 to 20 minutes. When curcumin is taken along with **bromelain**, it enhances the anti-inflammatory powers of bromelain and may be effective in relieving carpal tunnel syndrome.

How Does Turmeric Work?

The curcumin in turmeric appears to reduce pain by depleting the nerve endings of substance P, the neurotransmitter that carries pain receptors. As an anti-inflammatory, curcumin inhibits the formation of leukotrienes and the aggregation of platelets, dissolves blood clots and fibrin, and prevents the release of substances that cause inflammation.

Here's the Proof

In cases of acute inflammation, a comparison with the conventional drugs cortisone and phenylbutazone revealed that turmeric is as effective, but it is only half as effective in chronic inflammation. When researchers compared the effect of turmeric and phenylbutazone in patients with rheumatoid arthritis, both groups of patients had similar improvements in the amount of morning stiffness, joint swelling, and length of time they could walk. The advantage of using turmeric is the lack of side effects, which are significant with use of phenylbutazone.

How Safe Is Turmeric?
Turmeric is considered to be a safe herb that does not have any negative interactions with other remedies. Stomach upset may occur if you take dosages higher than those recommended. If you have gallstones, a blood-clotting disorder, or are pregnant, do not use turmeric unless under a doctor's care. Children and people older than 65 should take dosages below and up to the low end of the recommended dose range.

White Willow Bark

What Is White Willow Bark?
White willow bark (*Salix alba*) is a powerful natural pain reliever that is derived from the white willow tree. The Chinese have used it for its analgesic powers for centuries, but it was unknown to Western people until the eighteenth century. Many Native American

tribes were already using other species of the willow tree to treat fever, pain, and inflammation and as a wash for external ulcers when European settlers brought the white willow to the New World.

French and German scientists were the first to isolate salicin, the active ingredient in the willow, in 1828. A decade later, European chemists manufactured salicylic acid, a chemical similar to aspirin. This discovery eventually led to the creation of acetylsalicylic acid, our modern-day aspirin, although it was made from a different salicin-containing herb, meadowsweet.

White willow bark is just one of several willow tree species that are rich in salicin. The herbal remedy is made from the inner bark of the tree. You may also find crack willow (*Salix fragilis*), violet willow (*S. daphnoides*), bay willow (*S. pentandra*), and purple willow (*S. purpurea*) in health food stores, sold as willow bark rather than white willow bark.

What Types of Pain Does White Willow Bark Help?

- Back pain
- Burns (as a wash)
- Dysmenorrhea
- Headache and migraine
- Neuralgia
- Osteoarthritis
- Rheumatoid arthritis
- Sciatica

How Do You Use White Willow Bark?

White willow bark comes in capsule, tincture, and powder forms and as dried bark suitable for making a decoction. The preferred forms are capsules, tinctures, or powder standardized to contain 15 percent salicin. Decoctions are generally not very effective because they contain a very low percentage of salicin (usually around 1 percent). The infusion (cooled) can be helpful, however, as a wash for burns. Typical dosages are up to six 400-mg capsules or tablets daily or 10 to 30 drops tincture in water two to three times daily.

Many of the white willow supplements in the United States are not standardized. Be sure to buy only standardized supplements, as the percentage of salicin can vary widely, with some brands containing only minute amounts of the active ingredient.

Some health professionals suggest white willow for migraine relief. Unlike feverfew, which must be taken daily to help prevent a migraine attack, willow can be effective during an episode. Take 3 to 5 ml of tincture every two hours until the pain subsides.

How Does White Willow Bark Work?

Once salicin enters the body, it metabolizes in the liver and the blood to form salicylic acid, a substance that reduces inflammation, pain, and fever. White willow bark and other types of willow bark appear to suppress the action of prostaglandins, an action that reduces inflammation. Willow bark also contains other compounds that the body metabolizes to salicylic acid and therefore acts more slowly and maintains its pain-relieving benefit over a longer period than aspirin does. Willow also contains substances called tannins, which help reduce swelling.

Here's the Proof

There is some debate about the effectiveness of white willow bark for the treatment of pain and inflammation. Scientists agree that the herb contains salicin, yet they do not agree the levels are sufficient to provide adequate relief. In Germany, where white willow bark is highly endorsed and commonly used for arthritis, headache, and fever, the supplements are standardized, ensuring therapeutic levels. In the United States, however, standardized formulas are much harder to find.

How Safe Is White Willow Bark?

White willow bark is safe when used at the recommended doses. Some people, however, may experience an upset stomach, nausea, or ringing in the ears at higher doses. Unlike aspirin, it does not promote stomach bleeding. To help avoid stomach distress, Michael Tierra, author of *The Way of Herbs* and *Planetary Herbology*, suggests taking a small amount of cinnamon bark or licorice root with white willow bark. If you are allergic to aspirin or have ulcers or another type of gastrointestinal problem, do not take white willow bark. If you are pregnant or breastfeeding, ask your doctor before taking this herb. Children or teenagers who have a cold, flu, fever, or chicken pox should avoid using white willow bark because of its similarities to aspirin, which can cause Reye's syndrome, a potentially fatal disease, among this age group.

CHAPTER FIVE

Other Natural Approaches: Mind-Body Therapy and Energy Therapy

When you are hurting, how do you feel about the pain? Angry? Frustrated? Afraid? Helpless? Do you get tense, anxious, irritable, or impatient? If you are like most people, you tend to respond to pain in ways that make it worse. You deny it, resist it, hate it, even make bargains with God. But the secret to resolving pain is to stop wasting energy fighting it and start controlling it.

An integral part of using your mind and body to control chronic pain is to look at how you perceive pain. Psychiatrists, psychologists, and other mental health professionals stress that you need to realize that the pain is not a punishment; nor is it your fault, someone else's fault, or something that is beyond your control. If you have this negative or hopeless attitude about your pain, you make yourself a victim who is destined to suffer.

To use the mind-body connection successfully to control your pain, you need to "own" your pain. What this means is that you need to take responsibility—

not blame—for your pain, before you can control it. Responsibility means that you admit the pain is yours and accept it even though you don't want it. When you accept that the pain is part of you and that you can make conscious decisions about your behaviors, activities, and thoughts, then you can gain some control over it.

No one is sure exactly how the mind-body connection works. One popular theory, however, is offered by Ernest Rossi, author of *Psychobiology of Mind-Body Healing*. He explains that the mind-body connection reaches the cellular level and involves three stages, which include very complex biochemical reactions. In stage 1 the mind sends images deep into the brain to the cerebral cortex. In stage 2 the hypothalamus (the area of the brain that regulates involuntary actions such as breathing and blood pressure) processes the images and sends out neurotransmitters—chemicals such as serotonin and adrenaline—that carry messages which impact the autonomic nervous system. In stage 3 these neurotransmitters trigger changes in the body's functions, such as increasing production of the body's natural painkillers: endorphins, epinephrine (a stimulant), and norepinephrine (a relaxant).

Although the mechanisms of pain relief for mind-body techniques are not completely understood, they have caught the attention and approval of the conventional medical community. In 1996 a 12-member panel of medical experts from the National Institutes of Health convened. The NIH formed this panel to evaluate data on the treatment of chronic pain and insomnia because "to date, conventional medical and surgical approaches have failed, at considerable expense." After extensive study, they reported that "[we] found strong evidence for the use of relaxation techniques in reducing chronic pain in a variety of medical conditions." This report, published by the *Journal of the American Medical Association*, is the kind of endorsement mind-body medicine needed to convince the rest of the conventional medical community of what many in the general public know: that mind-body medicine works.

In this chapter you will learn about five different natural techniques that use the body-mind connection and the power of your body's energy to control pain. Biofeedback, hypnosis (self-hypnosis), meditation, and visualization/guided imagery are all mind-body techniques that, once mastered, will allow you to gain control over your pain. With the exception of biofeedback (which requires some equipment in the learning stages), you possess all you need to get the pain relief you want. With patience and practice, you can train your mind to be an analgesic—without side effects! Or you can draw upon your body's own energy field and learn to control your pain using magnets.

The best introduction to any mind-body or energy technique is breathing. Proper breathing is, in itself, a therapy that places people in a state of complete relaxation and helps control pain. Practice the breathing exercise described in the sidebar as a prelude to the exercises in this chapter. It can be done by anyone experiencing pain and/or who wants to reduce stress. Practice it at least twice a day and see if you don't notice a difference.

BREATHING EXERCISE

1. Place the tip of your tongue against the ridge behind and above your upper front teeth. Keep it there through the entire exercise.
2. Exhale completely through your mouth, making a "whoosh" sound as the air leaves you.
3. While keeping your mouth closed, inhale deeply and quietly through your nose to the count of 4.
4. Hold your breath for a count of 7.
5. Exhale through your mouth to a count of 8, making a "whoosh" sound.
6. Repeat steps, 3, 4, and 5 for a total of four breaths.

During the first month you practice this breathing exercise, do not do more than four breaths at one time, but practice as often as you wish. After a month, increase to eight breaths each time if you wish.

Biofeedback

What Is Biofeedback?
Biofeedback is a technique in which people use special instruments, learned procedures, or both to re-

ceive information from the body about what is happening within it. The word "biofeedback" means "living" (bio) feedback. This technique, which was developed in the United States in the 1970s, allows people to enhance the subtle messages that the body gives out so they can control or regulate those functions that cause or contribute to pain. People who master biofeedback can learn how to control their breathing rate, heart rate, blood circulation to specific parts of the body, body temperature, and muscle contractions.

What Types of Pain Does Biofeedback Help?

- Back pain
- Cancer pain
- Dysmenorrhea
- Headache and migraine
- Temporomandibular joint syndrome (TMJ)

Generally, biofeedback is effective for chronic rather than acute pain, because it usually takes several weeks to learn biofeedback techniques well enough that they will benefit you. Once learned, however, you can use them whenever you need to.

How Do You Use Biofeedback?

Most people learn biofeedback at a clinic or biofeedback center where they work with various types of biofeedback equipment. Once they master the techniques, though, the majority of people can practice biofeedback at home without the equipment. Many metropolitan areas have pain centers or teaching facilities that offer biofeedback, and some physicians have the equipment in their offices. (See Appendix A for help in locating a biofeedback center.)

For people with migraine and chronic severe headache, biofeedback is most effective when it is used as a preventive measure. When practiced daily, it significantly reduces the severity and frequency of headache and migraine. If you wait until you have a migraine attack, the results will be less powerful. People with chronic pain who practice biofeedback daily find it gives them a much-needed sense of control over their pain and an opportunity to live their lives more fully.

Biofeedback involves learning how to read your body's signals. To do that, you will learn to use one or more types of biofeedback machines, the most common of which is electromyographic (EMG) biofeedback. This type is most often used for tension headache and chronic muscle pain. The equipment includes a monitoring device that looks like a TV set. During each biofeedback session, you sit in a comfortable chair in front of the monitor. Several sensor wires with electrodes attached to them run from the machine to your body. The electrodes are taped to the skin over your painful areas. In order to get their muscles to relax, people often utilize other mind-body techniques, including visualization/guided imagery, hypnosis, and meditation. This marriage between biofeedback and other mind-body techniques is an excellent example of the complementary nature of natural remedies. Being attached to a biofeedback monitor while using one of these relaxation techniques provides a unique opportunity to gauge pain relief visually.

The electrodes send back (feedback) signals to the monitor, which measures the amount of electrical activity in the painful area. The feedback may be in the form of bleeps on the screen, graphic lines, or even audible beeps. After several sessions, you will have learned how to reduce pain and tension by using the feedback from the machine to help you visualize the pain so you can better control it. Then you will be able to practice at home without the machine.

Another type of biofeedback is thermal; people who want to relieve migraine pain often use thermal biofeedback. Here a sensor measures skin temperature, which is an indication of blood flow fluctuations. A characteristic of people with migraine is poor circulation, which leaves them with cold hands and feet. People with migraine can learn to increase the blood circulation in their hands and feet, which draws it away from their head and thus relieves the pressure in the blood vessels of the head. Most people who try this method can see a significant change in their temperature after four or five sessions and soon can get the same results without the machinery. Some people who are skilled at this biofeedback technique can warm their hands in just a few seconds.

Biofeedback is not an instant pain reliever: it requires patience, dedication, and practice. But the paybacks are great: reduction or elimination of painkillers and their associated side effects and cost and the freedom to alleviate your pain anytime, anywhere, once you've mastered the technique.

How Does Biofeedback Work?

Researchers have not defined exactly how biofeedback works. The results of some studies suggest it works because individuals make physical changes that lead to pain relief; for example, they can cause their blood vessels to expand and stimulate blood flow to the hands and feet and away from the head. But other studies show that many people experience significant or complete pain relief without demonstrating any physiological changes. Biofeedback may give them a sense of control over their pain and make them feel less helpless. It's been proven that when people feel they have the tools to take control of their pain, they are more motivated to work at eliminating it, and often they are successful.

Another explanation may lie with the fact that people in Western cultures tend to be more accepting of things they can see and measure. Pain is a subjective phenomenon and thus basically unmeasurable. Biofeedback allows people to "see" their pain, which makes it not only tangible and easier to manage but also validates it as real. It's also possible that biofeedback works due to a combination of these factors, plus others yet unknown. But for the tens of thousands of people for whom it provides relief, the "why" seems secondary.

Here's the Proof

In a 1990 issue of *Pain*, investigators reported on the results of more than 35 clinical studies that evaluated the effectiveness of biofeedback and relaxation training in reducing the frequency and severity of migraine. They found that when compared with the migraine drug Inderal (propranolol), the mind-body techniques were just as effective, plus there were no side effects. Other studies show that 75 percent of people with severe chronic headache experience relief from biofeedback.

Between 20 and 30 percent of people who suffer with migraine experience an aura phase before the pain begins. An aura phase is a 5- to 20-minute period during which a person has visual disturbances (e.g., spots or zigzag lines before the eyes, tunnel vision) and often a pins-and-needles sensation anywhere in the body. A review of 23 studies of the effectiveness of thermal biofeedback in patients who have migraine with aura shows that 52 percent have significant improvement if they practice biofeedback at the first sign of the aura.

Although anecdotal reports abound on the effectiveness of biofeedback for the relief of pain, very few scientific studies have been done on other types of pain besides headache and migraine. A few are worth noting. Several studies conducted by researchers in the United States, Sweden, and Holland report that between 40 and 60 percent of patients successfully treat TMJ pain with biofeedback. In a 1992 study reported in *Pain*, individuals with chronic back pain underwent 12 one-hour biofeedback sessions. Their results were compared with other patients who received bogus feedback (information from other patients). The patients who received the bona fide feedback had at least a 40 percent reduction in pain intensity, and half of these patients had a 75 percent decline in pain. The patients who received the bogus biofeedback reported no improvement in pain.

How Safe Is Biofeedback?

Biofeedback is a safe, noninvasive approach to pain relief. Many health care professionals recommend biofeedback to their patients as a complementary treatment for pain. Often it allows individuals to reduce or eventually eliminate any pain medications or other drugs they are taking as they become more adept at biofeedback. Let your physician know you are using biofeedback and consult with him or her before reducing your dosage of any medications. Also inform your biofeedback therapist about any medications you are taking.

Biofeedback devices are safe, and all but one do not conduct an electrical current. That one is the electrodermal machine, which measures changes in sweat activity and is used to treat anxiety. The amount of electricity transmitted cannot shock the recipient. As a safety precaution, the Association for Applied Psychophysiology and Biofeedback recommends that anyone who has a pacemaker or any other implanted electrical device or anyone with a serious heart disorder ask their physician before using this machine, although there have been no reports of any problems with the device.

Hypnosis

What Is Hypnosis?

Have you ever focused or concentrated on something so intently that you were not aware of what was going on around you? If you have, you've experienced hypnosis, a state of altered awareness that gives you an increased ability to respond to suggestions you give to yourself or someone else presents to you. Although the word "hypnosis" is derived from a Greek word for sleep, a hypnotic state is not one of drowsiness; it is one of intense, inwardly focused concentration. While in this changed mental state, you maintain your free will and your consciousness, which means you will not do anything that goes against your value system. Yet this altered mental state can allow you to significantly reduce or even eliminate your pain, relieve stress, and achieve greater emotional and spiritual peace. This section talks about self-hypnosis, which is an easy, safe, and effective way for you to hypnotize yourself, whenever you need to, without having to run to a hypnotherapist's office for a session.

Many people see similarities between self-hypnosis and guided imagery and between self-hypnosis and meditation, and indeed there are some. For example, in all three you are in an altered state of consciousness, and all can help you relieve pain using the power of your mind. A key difference among them is that in self-hypnosis, you tell yourself how you will achieve your goal; in guided imagery, you see yourself doing it and draw on your other senses to make the experience more powerful and complete; and with meditation, you clear the mind of images and concentrate on one word, thought, or action only. Each has its place in pain control, and each one has its own kind of appeal to different people.

What Types of Pain Does Self-hypnosis Help?

Virtually any type of pain can be relieved using self-hypnosis. According to Karen Olness, M.D., professor of family medicine at Case Western Reserve University, "Nearly every normal adult and child can use self-hypnosis to reduce the fear and anxiety that accompany pain and that can heighten it." Ninety-four percent of people who use hypnosis get some relief, even if it is only a reduction in stress, which in itself has a positive effect on pain. The type of pain and the degree it can be relieved are limited only by the extent to which you believe in the power of self-hypnosis and how much you are willing to practice. (See "How Does Self-Hypnosis Work?") Self-hypnosis has proven effective in treating the following types of pain. This does not mean you cannot try it to relieve other pain you may be experiencing:

- Burns
- Cancer pain

- Childbirth
- Headache and migraine
- Toothache

How Do You Use Self-Hypnosis?

You can learn self-hypnosis from a professional hypnotherapist or from a book, audiotape, or videotape. If you choose to learn self-hypnosis on your own, it is recommended that you take a session or two from a professional so you can better learn the techniques firsthand. It is important that you choose a hypnotherapist who is knowledgeable about the problem you want to remedy. Once you understand the basics, you can practice self-hypnosis anytime and without the expense of returning to a hypnotherapist.

The Biofeedback Certification Institute of America certifies hypnotherapists in the United States. More than 1,800 health professionals have received their credentials from the institute, although noncredentialed therapists also can be qualified to practice hypnotherapy by virtue of their experience. (See Appendix A for the institute's address.) According to the American Society of Clinical Hypnosis, more than 3,000 physicians, psychologists, and dentists incorporate hypnotherapy into their practice.

One form of self-hypnosis is autogenic training. This basic method, developed by Dr. Johannes Schultz in 1929, allows participants to reach a hypnotic state by repeating simple phrases while they focus on different parts of the body. It is an easy approach to pain management and a good exercise with which to start your self-hypnosis experience. Autogenic training can be learned from certified instructors or from self-help books. (See Bibliography and Suggested Reading.) Leon Chaitow, D.O., N.D., an author of several books, including *Holistic Pain Relief*, says that autogenics "comes close to duplicating the benefits of biofeedback without using machines." His experience shows that after about a month of practicing autogenics, people come very close to the same results they would get from using a biofeedback machine.

Before you try the autogenic exercise, read through the following guidelines:

•*Choose a comfortable location where you will not be disturbed for about 20 to 30 minutes. You will not always need this length of time; after you learn to enter a hypnotic state quickly, an entire session can last as little as 10 minutes. While you are learning, however, it often takes 15 minutes to reach a state of altered consciousness.*

•*Choose a position that is most comfortable for you. Because you are treating pain, your ability to relax as much as possible during a self-hypnosis session is of utmost importance.*

•*Most people close their eyes during a hypnotic session because it helps them focus. If keeping your eyes open works well for you, then do it.*

•*Proper breathing is critical for entering a hypnotic state. Refer to the "Breathing Exercise" on page 169 and do it before the Autogenic Exercise.*

AUTOGENIC EXERCISE

As you complete the breathing exercise, continue to breathe slowly and gently. As you breathe, repeat silently the phrase "I am at peace" until you feel completely relaxed.

Once you feel relaxed, repeat silently "My right arm is heavy." Repeat it several times while you concentrate on your right arm. Observe how your right arm feels, and notice any emotions or feelings that arise as you focus on your arm. There is no right or wrong way to feel; simply feel. If any other thoughts come to mind, allow them to leave and refocus on your arm.

Repeat silently, "My left arm is heavy." Again, repeat it several times while concentrating on your left arm and observe any emotions or feelings.

Do the same procedure for each of the following phrases:

"My right leg is heavy."

"My left leg is heavy."

"My arms and legs are heavy and warm."

"My heartbeat is calm and regular."

"My breathing is calm and regular."

"My center is warm."

"My forehead is cool."

"My neck and shoulders are heavy."

"I am _____ (give a personal affirmation, such as "I am in control of my pain" or "I am at peace with my pain").

For best results, practice this autogenic exercise twice a day. It is good as a general pain reliever. If your pain is associated with inflammation—arthritis, fibromyalgia, or bursitis, for example—replace the word "heavy" with "cool." Dr. Chaitow finds that this suggestion can reduce inflammation and pain in people with inflammatory conditions.

Once you become proficient at entering a hypnotic state, you'll be able to complete a session in about 10 minutes, short enough to do on your break at work. This simple mind-body technique can reduce pain, relieve tension and stress, and regulate blood and energy flow. It is a good introduction to self-hypnosis and prepares you for other sessions to treat specific painful conditions. The Bibliography and Suggested Reading List and Appendix A provide sources of self-hypnosis scripts and instructions.

How Does Hypnosis Work?

To best explain how hypnosis works, it helps to understand the type of person for whom it works best. If you agree with each of the following statements, you are probably a good candidate for self-hypnosis.

•*I have a good imagination.* Not only must you have a vivid imagination that includes all your senses, you must *believe* you have that power. According to Karen Olness, M.D., children are especially good at self-hypnosis because they usually have very good imaginations and are more willing than adults to try new things.

•*I am willing to take personal responsibility for relieving my pain.* Self-hypnosis allows you to take control of at least some of your pain. Pain relief using self-hypnosis does not happen overnight, however. It requires a firm commitment to practice every day.

•*I know what my goals are with self-hypnosis.* Set realistic goals and believe you can achieve them. If painful arthritis prevents you from gardening and you want to garden again, set that as your goal. Declaring you want to be completely pain free may be too unrealistic a goal. Define your goal clearly—write it down and put it on your refrigerator if you have to—so you can focus on it.

•*I am willing to devote the time it takes to learn and practice self-hypnosis.* It can take weeks or months of daily practice before you become proficient at self-hypnosis, but those who do say the payoff is great: pain control whenever they need it, and without drug side effects.

Each of these statements embodies the explanation of how hypnosis works: It works when people allow their mind to exercise its inherent power to control functions of the body. Self-hypnosis allows you to deliberately divert your attention away from your pain and refocus it onto imagery of your choosing. The process you use to refocus your attention places you in an altered state of consciousness. Then, once you are in a hypnotic state, you use the power of suggestion to reduce or eliminate pain.

You can choose whatever cue or suggestion you

wish. One woman who works as a cashier in a grocery store and who suffers with carpal tunnel syndrome, for example, gave herself the hypnotic suggestion that when she wears a blue blouse, her pain will subside. This works particularly well for her, especially since part of her required work attire is a blue blouse.

About 80 percent of people can be hypnotized: 20 percent are very susceptible, and 60 percent can be hypnotized to varying degrees. Only about 20 percent of people resist hypnosis, but they can be hypnotized too if they are willing to let down their resistance.

Here's the Proof

Hypnosis has been recognized by the conventional medical community as an effective treatment for pain. According to a 12-member panel of medical experts from the National Institutes of Health, hypnosis reduces several types of pain, including burn pain and lower back pain, by changing a person's perception of the pain. The panel also suggested that hypnosis can stop pain from entering consciousness through various brain functions, although exactly how pain is inhibited is not understood.

Self-hypnosis has proven especially beneficial in reducing migraine attacks among children and teenagers. At least 12 controlled studies have shown self-hypnosis to be the recommended approach for reducing the frequency and severity of migraine in young people. Similar studies have shown it to be helpful in adults as well. Other research shows that cancer pa-

tients undergoing chemotherapy experience little or
no nausea and less pain if they are hypnotized before
treatment. Burn patients who are hypnotized within
two hours of their injuries heal faster and with less
pain medication. Some investigators theorize that
these patients are able to heal more quickly because
they can influence the release of natural anti-
inflammatory factors.

How Safe Is Hypnosis?

Self-hypnosis is very safe, especially if you remember
that the myths surrounding hypnotism are just that—
pure fiction. All hypnosis is self-hypnosis, so no one
can "force" you to do anything against your will. Similarly, a hypnotic state is one of intense concentration,
not an unconscious state. Your attention is focused
inward instead of outward, but if something were to
occur in your environment that you needed to respond
to immediately, such as a fire, you would be completely aware of the danger.

There also is no danger of being "stuck" in a hypnotic state or forgetting the "secret ritual" to come
out of it. You are always in control and can come out
of a hypnotic state at any time.

Self-hypnosis can be used as the primary or a complementary treatment. It is recommended that you be
diagnosed by a medical professional for your health
problems before starting self-hypnosis. Also let him
or her know you are using hypnosis, especially if you
are taking medication, as it will likely reduce your

need for pain relievers once you become proficient at self-hypnosis.

Magnet Therapy

~~~~~

What Is Magnet Therapy?

In simple terms, magnet therapy is the use of magnets (like those on your refrigerator only much more powerful) to heal the body. Julian Whitaker, M.D., author of *The Pain Relief Breakthrough: The Power of Magnets*, explains that looking for "a simple, straightforward definition of magnetism" may cause people to become "a bit frustrated." So rather than define it, let's look at the big picture.

First, there is a close relationship between electricity and magnetism, which together form a key force in the universe called electromagnetism. Second, everything on Earth, living and nonliving, possesses electrical impulses, and all electrical impulses create a magnetic field. The human body—in particular the nervous system and the brain—depends on electrochemical impulses. Proof that there is electrical activity in the body is easy enough to see; consider, for example, that physicians use the electrocardiogram (ECG) to monitor the heart's electrical impulses. Similarly, the electromylogram (EMG) and electroencephalogram (EEG) record the activity of the skeletal muscles and the brain, respectively. Many scientists believe magnetic energy even is involved in stimulation of cell formation and division.

In any case, investigators know that magnetic energy, both within the body and external to it, has a significant impact on human health and well-being. Thus people—and their health—can be influenced by magnets and magnetism.

Magnetism: A Brief History. Modern civilizations were not the first to take advantage of the healing powers of magnets. Writings from the ancient Chinese, Egyptian, Greek, and other civilizations show that our ancestors used natural magnets to treat a variety of painful conditions. The ancient Greek Aristotle is believed to be the first person in recorded history to explain that magnets have therapeutic value. The medical system that the Chinese have used for more than 5,000 years is, in fact, based on bioelectricity: the flow of chi, or vital energy, through channels in the body known as meridians.

The man credited with introducing magnet therapy to Western medicine was born in 1493 in Switzerland. The alchemist, metallurgist, and physician Paracelsus was the first doctor to expand the use of magnets to treat conditions as diverse as diarrhea and epilepsy. In 1600 a mathematician named William Gilbert published a major work in which he proposed that the Earth was a magnet with magnetic poles at its northern- and southernmost extremes.

The person who is perhaps the most responsible for introducing magnets to the general population was Anton Mesmer. In 1775 he wrote *On the Medicinal Uses of the Magnet*, in which he described how he cured a patient of painful seizures and nervous system disorders using magnets. Mesmer believed that restoring the magnetic fields in the body was a requirement for health. Other researchers around the world continued to investigate both the curative properties of magnetism and the idea of magnetism as a science. In the 1800s magnet therapy increased in popularity as Benjamin Franklin conducted his experiments with electricity and searched for painless treatments for all sorts of medical conditions. As the year 1900 rolled around, the Sears Roebuck catalog was selling magnetic jewelry and magnetic boot soles. Medical textbooks discussed the use of magnet therapy and electricity to treat emotional and neurological conditions.

With the large influx of pharmaceuticals after World War II and the emphasis on medical and surgical procedures, magnet therapy was pushed aside in the United States. Elsewhere, however, interest in magnet therapy continued. More than 45 countries now have officially recognized magnet therapy as a medical treatment, while in the United States it has gained acceptance outside the medical arena.

Types of Magnet Therapy. Two types of magnets—electromagnets and permanent magnets—are used in magnet therapy. Electromagnets are produced when an electric current flows between a coil of wire called a solenoid. This type of magnetic field can be turned on and off and is often referred to as pulsed electromagnetism. It is the type of magnetism used to perform ECGs and magnetic resonance imaging (MRI) as well as to help heal fractures. Pulsed electromagnetism requires expensive equipment, visits to a treatment facility, and trained personnel to do the therapy. Although it plays a key role in health, it is not practical for self-treatment of pain.

Permanent magnets are pieces of metal that possess magnetic energy. Various materials are used to make magnets; a combination of one-fifth boron and four-fifths neodymium makes the most powerful magnet. A mixture of aluminum, iron, cobalt, copper, and nickel (alnico) magnets is ten times more powerful than steel magnets; ferrite magnets, composed of carbonates of barium and iron, are more powerful than alnico magnets, but are very brittle.

A magnet's magnetic field is created by the movement of electrons within the material that makes it up. When it comes to treating pain, especially self-treatment, permanent magnets are the clear choice. They are readily available, affordable, simple to use, and, most important, effective in relieving or eliminating pain.

What Types of Pain Does Magnet Therapy Help?
Scientific studies of the effectiveness of magnet therapy on pain is in its infancy. Clinical studies conducted thus far show magnets can be beneficial in the treatment of:

• Back pain
• Bursitis and tendinitis
• Cancer pain

- Carpal tunnel syndrome
- Dysmenorrhea
- Fibromyalgia
- Headache
- Muscle pain
- Osteoarthritis
- Rheumatoid arthritis

Because magnet therapy is a relatively new field, there are as many questions as there are answers. Scientists have yet to uncover which kinds of magnets work best for different kinds of pain or why they work for some people and not for others. It is hoped that answers to these and other questions will be found in the near future as research continues. Even the NIH is investigating the effectiveness of magnets. Two studies supported by the NIH's Office of Alternative Medicine—one on the ability of magnet mattress pads to reduce the pain of fibromyalgia and the other on whether magnets can help prevent stroke—are among the many currently under way around the world.

How Do You Use Magnet Therapy?
The strength of a magnet's magnetic field is measured using a unit called *gauss*, named after Carl Friedrich Gauss, a nineteenth-century German mathematician and physicist. The gauss number refers to the number of lines of magnetic force that pass through an area measuring 1 square centimeter. So before you go and yank the magnets off the door of your refrigerator, you should know that they aren't quite strong enough

for therapeutic purposes—they are only about 10 gauss. The gauss strength needed to treat pain depends on the type of pain, but most permanent magnets have a gauss number in the range of 400 to several thousand.

HOW TO BUY MAGNETS: TERMS TO KNOW

Choosing a permanent magnet to treat pain requires a bit of knowledge about a few terms. *Saturation magnetization* refers to the ultimate amount of magnetic field a magnet can produce. The higher the number, the better the magnetic field. A permanent magnet made of the best materials would have a saturation magnetization of about 15,000 gauss.

A permanent magnet also has *coercivity*, which is a measure of just how permanent a magnet is. The coercivity and saturation magnetization values together form an index called the *maximum energy product*, which is the measurement to look for when shopping for therapeutic permanent magnets. The maximum energy product is measured in units of gauss-oersted (Goe).

Magnets also have *North Pole* and *South Pole energy*. The north side of a magnet projects negative energy and has the properties of dispersing and inhibiting, which makes it the choice for treatment of pain. The physiological effects of magnets listed under "How Does Magnet Therapy Work?" are the result of North

Pole energy on the body. The South Pole has a positive force, which promotes growth and pro-liferation and is used, for example, to stimulate the immune system. When buying a magnet to treat pain, never buy one that has both the North and South energy poles on the same side (called a bipole magnet).

Buying a Medical Magnet. Medical magnets come in a wide range of strengths, sizes, shapes, and prices. For as little as $5 you can purchase a coin-shape magnet, or you can spend $900 or more for a magnetic mattress. The most reasonable and effective type of magnet to start with is a neodymium-boron magnet. Gauss strengths start as low as 100, and the range used for most painful conditions is 450 to 2,500. Buy your magnets from a company that offers a money-back guarantee of at least 30 days. Magnets do not work for everyone, although most people do experience at least some pain relief.

Once You Get the Magnet Home. If possible, consult with a knowledgeable professional about how to use your magnets. (See Appendix for information sources.)

To use a magnet, position it (or them if using more than one) over the painful area and secure it with medical adhesive tape or an Ace bandage. Be sure the north side is down against or facing the skin. If you are treating carpal tunnel syndrome, for example, you can place the magnets on your wrist and wrap the wrist with a bandage. People with foot pain often place the magnets in their shoes. For back pain, you can place coin-shape magnets on the skin or place block magnets under your mattress.

You can eliminate the need to tape and bandage magnets in place by using one of the many magnet products on the market. Magnetic seat cushions, jewelry, wristbands, shoe insoles, elbow and knee supports, mattresses, and other items are available from many different suppliers. (See Appendix B.) Always ask for the gauss or Goe of the magnet or magnet product you are buying to be sure you are getting sufficient magnetic power.

How Does Magnetic Therapy Work?

"There remains no reasonable doubt that all living organisms are extraordinarily sensitive to magnetic fields." So report Drs. Barnwell and Brown of the Department of Biological Sciences, Northwestern University. They, along with scientists around the world, continue to investigate the relatively new field of biomagnetics—how magnetism affects health and well-being.

Because every atom in nature generates an electromagnetic field, we, along with all animate and inanimate objects on Earth, have the power of electromagnetism; that is, we are biomagnetic. Researchers believe that permanent magnets, when applied to parts of the body, interact with the biomagnetic force of the body and can bring it into harmony and balance, health and healing. This healing appears to occur at both the cellular and subatomic levels. Some proponents of biomagnetics go a bit further with this line of thinking and say that health is based on the body's cells vibrating at a specific frequency. The presence of abnormal vibrations represents disease or imbalance. The application of magnets, therefore, restores normal cellular vibration.

Although no one is certain exactly how magnetic therapy works, researchers have come up with several viable theories. Many investigators, including Dr. Whitaker, believe there is more than one answer to the question "How does magnetic therapy work?" because biomagnetics works through a number of different mechanisms.

For example, scientific research has documented the following physiological effects of electromagnetism or magnetism on the body, all of which can have a positive effect on pain:

1. Magnetism increases blood flow and the circulation of oxygen and nutrients in the bloodstream. When a magnet is held against or near the skin, several things are thought to occur. The energy relaxes the capillary walls, thus stimulating blood flow. And because cells contain both positive and negative charges, they assume the polarity (magnetic pull) of the magnetic field that surrounds it. Thus the North Pole energy pulls oxygen into the cell. The increase in blood, oxygen, and nutrients that flow to damaged tissue reduces inflammation and swelling, carries away toxins, and thus reduces pain.

2. Magnetic therapy affects the pineal gland, which in turn stimulates production of various enzymes and the hormones melatonin and serotonin. There is a clear cause-and-effect relationship between each of these substances and pain, especially serotonin and pain. (See **5-HTP**.)

3. Application of magnets interferes with muscle contractions, thereby preventing the muscle spasms that are associated with many types of pain.

4. Magnetism appears to affect the electrochemical reactions that occur within nerve cells, thus interfering with their ability to send pain signals to the brain.

5. Magnets help normalize the pH balance, which is often out of balance (too acidic) in the presence of disease or illness, such as allergies, toxic states, sore muscles, and pain.

6. Magnetism speeds up the elimination of calcium ions from bones and nerve tissue and the buildup of calcium seen in arthritic joints.

More explanations are under investigation, though as yet there is limited experimental documentation to back them up. One theory speculates that magnets change the ability of the cells to conduct electricity by realigning certain molecules in the cell membranes. Another proposes that magnetism hinders the accumulation of the enzyme cholinesterase, which in turn inactivates a chemical responsible for pain control.

The fact that experts know that permanent magnets work yet don't understand why is not unusual in the world of medicine and healing. In fact, scientists are not completely sure why many of the drugs currently on the market work. Permanent magnets have clear advantages over drugs—the lack of annoying, often debilitating or dangerous side effects and the fact that they work so well. As more and more research is performed and the findings are made public, we are sure to find out how magnets work to reduce and eliminate pain—and discover their other benefits as well.

Here's the Proof

Many studies have proven the effectiveness of electromagnetism as a healer—for skin ulcers, fractures, damaged nerves, torn cartilage, wounds, soft-tissue damage, and tumors—and relief or elimination of headache, neck and back pain, arthritis, tendinitis, and other painful conditions. The success of these studies and the large number of anecdotal reports of pain relief from use of permanent magnets have prompted more scientific, controlled investigations into the use of permanent magnets for pain. Use and endorsement of magnets among professional athletes (e.g., pro golfers Arnold Palmer, Greg Norman, and Lisanne DiNapoli; members of the Miami Dolphin football team; speed skater Bonnie Blair; Denver Broncos linebacker Bill Romanowski) have helped thrust this pain remedy into the spotlight.

Research studies have been convincing as well.

Women with painful menstruation who took part in a placebo-controlled study at Seoul University reported significant pain reduction when magnets were applied over the pubic region. Ronald Lawrence, M.D., clinical professor of medicine at the University of California at Los Angeles, studied use of permanent magnets on patients with carpal tunnel syndrome. Nearly 90 percent of his patients experienced significant improvement after wearing the magnets for just one week.

The chronic pain experienced by many people with postpolio syndrome can be relieved by applying magnets at 300 to 500 gauss, according to a study conducted at the Baylor College of Medicine in Texas. Ninety percent of the more than 11,000 patients treated at Tokyo's Isuzu Hospital for muscle spasm in the neck and shoulder have gotten relief from use of magnet therapy. Another study in Japan reported that 90 percent of patients with bursitis, arthritis, and rheumatism had pain relief within five days of using magnets compared with only 14 percent of patients who were not treated with them.

How Safe Is Magnet Therapy?

Experts tell us that magnets are safe and, in fact, necessary. Magnetism holds our world together. The planet Earth has a magnetic field of half a gauss; your car has hundreds of magnets; and every electrical appliance in your home has at least one magnet in it. Scientists are always skeptical, however, and continue to investigate the safety of permanent magnets. So far, they conclude that the low gauss levels used with permanent magnets pose no health risks. Even levels as high as 15,000 gauss (from exposure to MRI machines) do not present a health hazard, explains Dr. Lawrence, although you would not want to be exposed to that strength for any length of time. According to experts on magnet therapy, permanent magnets of 2,500 gauss or less are completely safe regardless of which side (north or south) is used. It is believed that a small percentage of people may experience a minor imbalance if they are exposed to a high-level magnetic field (more than 3,000 gauss) for a prolonged period of time. Exposure to 3,000 gauss or higher should be limited to 30 minutes once or twice a day.

As with any form of therapy or medication, magnetic therapy should not be started without first consulting with your health practitioner. If you have unexplained pain, it is recommended that you determine the cause before attempting to treat it. Women who are pregnant, or anyone who is taking medication, has heart disease (especially a pacemaker), or has a chronic disease should not start magnet therapy without first talking with their physician.

Meditation

What Is Meditation?

Meditation, according to Bernie Siegel, M.D., who has done extensive research on meditation's benefits in the medical field, is "an active process of focusing the mind into a state of relaxed awareness," with the goal being to achieve a restful trance that frees and strengthens the mind. During meditation, you unclutter your mind, allowing images and thoughts that enter your consciousness to leave without acting upon them, unlike guided imagery and self-hypnosis, during which you would follow through on images and thoughts.

The two basic approaches to meditation are mindfulness and concentrative. Each form has many variations, but an understanding of the basics of both can help you get started and then move on to other levels as you wish.

Mindfulness Meditation. Mindfulness, or insight meditation, is a state of consciousness in which you allow yourself to be aware of the thoughts, sensations, and feelings that pass through your mind without allowing yourself to think about them. Joan Borysenko, Ph.D., author of *The Power of the Mind to Heal* and *Mind the Body, Mending the Mind*, calls these thoughts a "continuously passing parade of sensations and feelings." Jon Kabat-Zinn, Ph.D., director of the Stress Reduction Clinic at the University of Massachusetts Medical Center in Worcester, emphasizes that the key to mindfulness is "the quality of the awareness that you bring to each moment." Mindfulness is about being fully aware in the present moment. If you have physical pain, mindfulness meditation helps you see it as it is and to accept it. When you open up and become accepting, says Dr. Kabat-Zinn, you can become better able to respond more effectively to your situation.

During mindfulness meditation, thoughts often creep into the mind. When they do, let them float away without acting on or thinking about them. This takes practice and is not meant to frustrate you. Even the most practiced of meditators have intruding thoughts and have learned to simply let them pass by.

Concentrative Meditation. Concentrative meditation is the technique studied in the 1970s by Drs. Herbert Benson and R. Keith Wallace, who proved scientifically that this approach can reduce heart rate, oxygen use, and breathing rate after only a few weeks of practice. This type of meditation involves focusing on a repetitive sound, action, or image, which helps people quiet their mind and heighten awareness. Repetition of the humming sound "ohmmmmmmm," commonly referred to as a mantra, is perhaps one of the most common meditative focuses. Many people focus on their breathing, a flickering candle or fire in a fireplace, or a beautiful object. If you choose to do concentrative meditation for pain, choose a focus that is most relaxing and pleasing to you.

What Types of Pain Does Meditation Help?

As with other types of mind-body techniques, the types of pain you can relieve using meditation are limited primarily by the extent to which you believe in the power of meditation and how much you are willing to practice it. (See "How Does Meditation Work?") Dr. Borysenko notes that meditation is truly a mind-body experience, which is apparent by the fact that when people stop meditating, the physical benefits they gained tend to disappear within a few weeks.

Because meditation is primarily a relaxation technique, conditions associated with stress that involve pain, such as tension headache, respond best. People with chronic pain conditions (e.g., fibromyalgia and cancer pain) who have not responded completely to conventional medical treatment often get significant relief when using meditation as a complement to their other therapy.

The following conditions typically respond to meditation when practiced regularly. That does not mean meditation will not relieve other types of pain. With dedicated practice, meditation can help people with chronic pain get a new perspective on their condition and not allow their pain to control them. Meditation can alleviate their fears and feelings of helplessness and hopelessness, and give them a sense of spiritual well-being, which can improve their quality of life.

- Back pain
- Cancer pain
- Dysmenorrhea
- Fibromyalgia
- Headache
- Irritable bowel syndrome
- (PMS) Premenstrual syndrome
- Postsurgical pain
- Temporomandibular joint syndrome
- Ulcers

How Do You Use Meditation?

Ideally, meditation should be part of a daily routine. People who practice it daily report they are better able to manage their pain, feel more relaxed and rested, and can accomplish more during the day. How often you meditate depends on you and the type and severity of pain you want to control. Some people find that 15 minutes first thing in the morning and another 15 minutes before they retire provide the relief to get through the day and get to sleep at night. A 15-minute meditation at midday is just the boost others need to feel good for the rest of the day.

To prepare for a meditative session, many people find it helpful to get into a meditation pose. (See the sidebar.) If you have pain that does not allow you to get into this position, use any position that is most comfortable for you.

MEDITATION POSE

- Sit on the floor with your legs straight out in front of you and form a V shape.
- Bend your right leg and bring it toward you. Place the side of your right foot on the floor close to your groin.
- Bend your left leg and place your left foot on the floor close to your right leg.
- Rest your hands on your knees, arms outstretched and palms up.
- Keep your back straight.

Below are two exercises—one is an example of mindfulness, the other of concentrative meditation. You can tape these scripts so they will be conveniently at hand when you want to practice. You also can record meditation scripts from other books, purchase prerecorded meditations, or, in some cases, borrow them from your public library. (See Appendix B for sources.)

Mindfulness Meditation

•*Get into a comfortable position, lying down if possible. Use whatever pillows or cushions you need.*

•*Stretch slowly and fully so you feel completely present in your body. As you stretch, take an inventory of your body. Start with your toes and move up your body, acknowledging each body part's presence in your mind. When you reach a part that is painful, simply acknowledge the pain without making any judgment about it. Continue your inventory until you reach the top of your head.*

•*Close your eyes if they aren't closed already and take a deep, slow breath. Exhale fully and slowly.*

•*As you take your next deep breath, focus your attention on the spot just below your navel. For a moment or two, concentrate on sending each breath to that spot. Be aware as each breath arrives and leaves that spot, slowly and gently.*

•*Now allow yourself to shift your attention away from that spot and to become fully aware of your body. Focus on the spot that is painful. If more than one spot is a problem, concentrate on one spot and deal with it completely before you move on to another one.*

•*Send your breath to the painful site. As you inhale, be aware of any sensations in or around the spot. Simply be aware of the sensations without judging them or thinking about them. They are not good or bad, they simply are.*

•*As you exhale, notice if the sensations change. Allow your breath to sweep over the painful area as it leaves your body. Acknowledge any sensations and let them be. Continue to breathe in and out, slowly and gently, acknowledging any sensations that come to you. Stay with that site until you feel some relief.*

•*If you have another spot that needs attention, shift your breath to it. Repeat the process above.*

•*When you have addressed all the sites you wish to focus on, take several deep breaths, release them slowly, and open your eyes as you return to full consciousness.*

It may take you several sessions before you get significant pain relief. You also may experience a temporary increase in pain or discomfort. This occurs because you are focusing your attention on it. This discomfort usually decreases or even disappears as you continue to meditate.

Concentrative Meditation
•*Choose the meditation pose as described in the sidebar, or get into a position that is most comfortable for you.*

•*Close your eyes and allow your body to relax. If you are sitting, lift your chest and let your chin fall lightly toward your throat. Place your hands on your knees, palms up. If you choose, create a circle by bringing together the tips of your thumb and index finger of each hand.*

•*Inhale deeply and slowly through your nose. Hold the breath for a few seconds and then slowly exhale. Repeat this cycle for about two minutes. At the end of each exhale, squeeze your buttocks and hold this position for a few seconds. Concentrate only on your breath and the squeeze.*

•*After two minutes, switch your focus to anyplace in your body that is painful. Meditate on that spot and focus on sending your breath deeply into it. See that spot clearly in your mind. Continue to meditate on that spot and breathe deeply for about two minutes.*

•*If you have another painful site, switch your focus to that place and repeat the cycle in the last step.*

How Does Meditation Work?

When you meditate, your body enters an altered state of calm and peacefulness, one in which there are physical changes that can have a significant impact on pain. Scientific studies have shown, for example, that meditation lowers the level of stress hormones in the blood, reduces heart and breathing rates, lowers blood pressure, and brings down blood sugar levels. All of these reactions are part of the "relaxation response," a state of being in which the mind is cleared of thoughts and activity and settles into a state of restful, heightened awareness. (See works by Herbert Benson and Jon Kabat-Zinn in the Bibliography and Suggested Reading List.) Scientists have proven this state of relaxation exists by monitoring the brain waves of people who meditate. What they see is an increase in alpha brain wave activity, the brain waves that are present during states of deep relaxation and creativity.

Meditation also has a spiritual component, and for many people this is an integral part of their ability to reduce pain. The spiritual strength they gain from meditating allows them better to accept, deal with, and control their pain and its causes.

Dr. Borysenko believes the intruding thoughts that occur during mindfulness meditation actually serve a productive purpose by strengthening your "mental muscles of awareness and choice." Flexing these mental muscles is especially helpful for dispelling thoughts and sensations of pain. Each time you send pain sensations away, you exercise control over your pain and take back control of your life.

Here's the Proof
Proof of the benefits of meditation for the control and management of pain does not come from controlled clinical studies as much as it does from the results reported by participants in stress reduction clinics and programs around the country. Dr. Kabat-Zinn has had more than 6,000 patients go through the Stress Reduction Clinic's meditation program. Many thousands

more have attended similar clinics across the United States. Dr. Kabat-Zinn finds that "mindfulness . . . can improve a range of physical symptoms; reduce pain, depression, and anxiety; . . . and motivate patients to take better care of their health." Controlled scientific studies of meditation and its role in pain relief and healing are in the beginning stages.

How Safe Is Meditation?

Meditation is a safe, noninvasive way to control pain. It can be used as the primary or a complementary treatment, depending on the type of pain you wish to treat. It is recommended that you be diagnosed by a medical professional for your health problems before you start meditation. Most of the patients who attend Dr. Kabat-Zinn's clinic have been referred by their physicians, evidence of the credibility this form of mind-body approach has gained from the conventional medical arena. Inform your healthcare professional that you are using meditation, especially if you are taking medication, as you may be able to reduce your dosage as you become more experienced in meditation.

Visualization and Guided Imagery

What Are Visualization and Guided Imagery?

Visualization is a method of using one or more mental visual images (the "mind's eye") to achieve a specific goal such as to: relax, relieve stress; connect with your feelings or emotions; or to heal physical and/or emotional pain, disease, or discomfort. When you use guided imagery, you take visualization several steps beyond visual images and bring all of your senses into play: sound, smell, taste, and touch as well as sight. Then you use those images and senses to create scenarios in your mind—a mind-play if you will—that support your goal.

According to Belleruth Naparstek, author of *Staying Well with Guided Imagery: How to Harness the Power of Your Imagination for Health and Healing*, guided imagery is "a form of self-hypnosis that uses for its content the deliberate production of healing sensory images," Thus in order for guided imagery to be effective, you need to place yourself in an altered state of consciousness. This altered state is one of the key factors to why guided imagery works. (The term "guided imagery" will be used throughout this section, as it encompasses visualization.)

There are many approaches you can take to guided imagery, and several are very effective in dealing with pain. For example, in cellular imagery you focus on your body's activities at the cellular level. This requires that you have a basic understanding of the condition you want to treat, such as how the cells operate to cause inflammation. Physiological imagery also requires that you know a little about what is creating your pain so you can "see" how to fix it. Unlike cellular imagery, this type deals with life-size processes rather than microscopic ones. Perhaps the most popular and commonly used forms of guided imagery are the metaphoric model, in which you use symbols to deal with your issues, and the favorite-place, or feeling-state imagery. Very often people use favorite-place imagery and incorporate metaphors into their scenes to get a more powerful response to their sessions.

What Type of Pain Does Guided Imagery Help?

Because guided imagery is a cumulative therapy—its effects accumulate gradually over time and with regular practice—it can be very effective with chronic pain. However, the type of pain that can be helped with guided imagery is limited only by your imagination and commitment to practice. Therefore, most of the conditions listed may respond to guided imagery.

- Cancer pain
- Fibromyalgia
- Osteoarthritis
- Postsurgical pain
- Rheumatoid arthritis

How Do You Use Guided Imagery?

Anyone who is open to the powers of the mind and is willing to welcome those powers can learn to produce healing, healthy sensory images to relieve pain. Guided imagery allows you to interrupt your thoughts of denial, anger, and resistance to pain and to embrace it as a friend that needs comforting and love.

If you are feeling unsure or uneasy about practicing guided imagery or if you have difficulty imagining how to reduce or eliminate pain using your mind, try answering these questions. They are designed to help you experience your pain on more than one level and essentially give you a different perspective.

1. What color is your pain? Colors stimulate emotions and feelings.
2. What texture is your pain—hard, sharp, nagging, smooth, burning?
3. What images come to mind when you think about your pain? One woman said there was a fire raging in your stomach; another described her pain as being crushed by a heavy boulder.

Once you've better defined your pain, you need to imagine the healthy areas around the pain. This may seem difficult as well because even a small area of pain seems to take over the rest of the body. However, if you draw a simple figure of yourself and circle the area that hurts, you can visualize all the areas that do not. These painless areas are your healing zones, the areas of healthy tissue that can help transform the painful tissue. Many people find that the most effective images to relieve or eliminate pain are soothing, gentle ones in which the pain evaporates, melts, flies, fades, or blows away.

Guided Imagery Exercise
Feel free to expand on this simple exercise by making it longer or adding features that best suit your needs.

•*Choose a location where you will not be disturbed for 10 to 20 minutes and where the temperature and noise level are pleasant for you. Sit in a comfortable chair or choose another position in which you are most comfortable. Depending on where you hurt, lying down on your back or side or even standing may be best suited for you. Allow your body to relax as much as possible. Close your eyes and keep them closed throughout the session.*

•*Breathe in slowly to a count of 5 and then out slowly to a count of 5. Do this several times.*

•*Tighten the muscles in your toes to a slow count of 4 and then release.*

•*Tighten the muscles in your calves to a slow count of 4 and then release.*

•*Continue to work your way slowly up your body, tightening your muscles at each location to a slow count of 4 and then releasing—your thighs, buttocks, abdomen, forearms, shoulders, face, and neck. Continue to breathe deeply and slowly.*

•*As you breathe in, imagine you are breathing in the present and breathing out the past, releasing pain, worries, fears. Notice any sensations in your hands, feet, arms, neck, shoulders, and legs as you breathe in and out—any tingling, feelings of warmth, and release of tension.*

•*Now picture a place where you feel safe, secure, and at peace. It can be anyplace you've always wanted to go, or a place you've been before where you feel comfortable. It can be a real place or an imaginary one; it doesn't matter.*

•*Allow yourself to enter that place, be a part of it. . . . Let every sound fill your ears . . . inhale every smell and identify them. . . . If there are things to taste, do so with gusto.*

•*Look around you and notice every color, every shade and hue. . . . Reach out in your mind's eye and touch every object. Notice its texture, its warmth or coolness, its softness or hardness. . . .*

•*Feel the air on your skin or the sun on your shoulders or whatever surrounds you in the place you have chosen. Surrender yourself to the richness of your special place and the comfort it can bring.*

•*Take a deep breath and allow the peace and beauty of your special place to enter your body . . . feel it reach into every cell of your being . . . washing through you with gentle warmth and softness.*

•*Allow that peace and beauty to reach the place that holds the pain . . . feel as they surround the pain and soften it. Breathe into the pain and allow your breath to soften the pain. As you breathe out, allow pieces of the pain to gently leave your body, floating out on your breath.*

•*Breathe in again . . . and breathe out . . . allowing another bit of pain to leave. If you can, place your hands over the painful spot. Imagine your hands are lifting out the pain . . . allowing your breath to carry it away. . . .*

•*Continue to breathe in deeply and exhale easily, knowing that a piece of your pain leaves on every breath out . . . Know that as you gently release your pain, you are safe and secure in your special place*

... that it is a healing place, always within you and within your control. Know that with each deep breath you inhale healing energy ... that with each exhale you release pain. ...

•Knowing you can always return to this safe, healing place ... whenever you choose to ... you bid it farewell as you continue to breathe in and out slowly and easily ... gradually returning to the place you traveled from ... slowly opening your eyes when you are ready ... feeling energized and more in control and that you possess wonderful healing energy within you.

Here are some guidelines to consider when using guided imagery.

•You may use an audiotape of an imagery exercise or create one of your own using the script above or one from books available on the market (see Bibliography and Suggested Reading List). Tapes are a good way to get your imagination flowing, although some people find they can forgo a tape and create their own scenes.

•Relief from chronic pain will likely take time: experts recommend practicing imagery for ten to twenty minutes a day, once or twice a day, for three to four weeks before you can expect significant results.

How Does Guided Imagery Work?

The mind is a very powerful tool, and it has an incredible influence over the workings of the human body. According to Belleruth Naparstek, guided imagery is effective because of three factors. One is that the body can't clearly distinguish between what's real and what's imaginary if the sensory images are evocative. If you doubt it, try this simple experiment. Close your eyes and picture a lemon. Now see yourself cutting the lemon in half with a knife and placing half of the lemon into your mouth. Imagine you are sucking on the lemon. Are your lips puckering up involuntarily? Can you taste the sourness of the lemon? You have just used a simplified form of guided imagery, using sight, feel, and taste. Simple, yet powerful.

The second reason refers back to the idea of being in an altered state of consciousness. When people put themselves into a relaxed, highly focused state of calm alertness, as in a hypnotic state, they have an increased capacity to heal, change, and learn. Several of the ways to achieve this state of heightened calm and awareness were discussed in "How Do You Use Guided Imagery."

The third factor that makes guided imagery successful is that people naturally feel better about themselves when they feel they have control over what is happening to them. Many people in pain feel they are helpless to do anything to improve their situation, especially if they suffer with chronic pain. This perceived lack of control contributes to feelings of hopelessness and low self-esteem. These feelings can have negative effects on all areas of people's lives, even to the point of destroying their ability to work, socialize, and maintain relationships.

According to Norman J. Marcus, M.D., author of *Freedom from Chronic Pain*, "when you tap into your imagination, you discover the very individual images you associate with causing pain and with stopping pain." The images and scenes you create in your mind when you are in a highly relaxed state "are a highly personalized prescription for eliminating pain."

Here's the Proof

Few well-controlled studies of the medical benefits of guided imagery have been done. However, countless clinical and anecdotal reports show that it is helpful in the treatment of various chronic pain conditions and stress-related ailments. Innovative work with imagery was done in the early 1970s by O. Carl Simonton, a radiation oncologist, and Stephanie Simonton, a psychologist, who taught cancer patients to use guided imagery to fight their disease. Although no controlled studies show that patients made their tumors shrink or disappear, some doctors and patients claim it has happened. More often, however, patients report relief from pain and anxiety and a feeling of control over their disease.

In a one-year study conducted by David Spiegal, a psychiatrist at Stanford University, 86 women with breast cancer were divided into two groups. All the women received the same medical treatment, yet one group also learned to use self-hypnosis and guided imagery to help them relieve pain, tension, and stress.

At the end of the study, the women who had used guided imagery said they had much less pain and discomfort, a greater feeling of control and well-being, and fewer mood swings. In addition, the group that used guided imagery also lived an average of twice as long as the other group

How Safe Is Guided Imagery?

In most situations, guided imagery is very safe. Do not use it in place of necessary medical treatment or while operating a car or machinery. Because imagery can change your body's need for medications, consult with your physician before you start using guided imagery. Do not stop taking any prescribed medications on your own without first talking with your doctor.

CHAPTER SIX

Buying and Using Natural Pain Relievers

In the introduction, you were told that this book would show you three easy steps to natural pain relief: (1) learning about the condition you want to treat and which natural pain relievers are recommended; (2) learning all you need to know about the remedies that are recommended; and (3) buying and using the remedy. This chapter helps you with step 3. The "How Do You Use" section in each of the entries in Chapters 4 and 5 outlined the specific remedies, dosages, and how to take them for specified conditions. This chapter covers general instructions for buying and using herbal and homeopathic remedies and natural supplements.

Which Form Is Best?

Unless the "How Do You Use" instructions specify which form is best to treat your condition (e.g., capsaicin cream for osteoarthritis), you may have to choose between tablet or capsule, extract or decoction, powder or liquid. For any given supplement, usually at least one form is more effective than another. To help you make a choice, follow these guidelines:

•*Some herbal supplements are labeled as "standardized" extracts, or "guaranteed potency extract." This means that the extract is guaranteed to contain a predetermined, or standardized, level of active ingredients. Because supplements are not regulated by the Food and Drug Administration, consumers cannot be certain they are getting the potency listed on a supplement's packaging. With standardized supplements, manufacturers assure consumers that the product contains a guaranteed amount of active ingredient. Knowing the level of active components allows you to take more accurate dosages. Thus you are more likely to get the benefits you desire.*

•*In herbal medicine, standardized forms are usually superior to all other forms. Solid extracts, fluid extracts, and tinctures are generally more potent than are infusions, decoctions, or powdered herbs. Capsules may contain standardized leaves, powder, or another form of the herb, but the label should state that the contents are standardized.*

•*When taking any remedy or supplement, consider your needs and lifestyle. Some people have difficulty swallowing tablets and capsules, especially elderly adults and people with various medical conditions. Sprays, tinctures, extracts, and powders may be best in these cases. If the supplement you need is available in tablets and capsules only, ask your pharmacist or physician if breaking a tablet into halves or quarters or sprinkling the contents of a capsule into liquid will change the effectiveness of the remedy.*

•If a remedy or supplement is equally effective in several forms, the one you choose may simply be a matter of convenience or preference. Some people prefer a tincture or extract so they can add it to a glass of juice in the morning and evening; others travel a lot and find that tablets are most convenient.

•Some supplements have fillers called excipients—nonnutritional ingredients that help hold the supplement together. They are found most often in tablets and capsules. If you have a food allergy or food sensitivity, be aware of the fillers and other added ingredients that may be in the remedy you've chosen. Many products are available that are free of yeast, milk, salt, soy, corn, starch, sugar, and wheat. Look on the packaging for information about additives and fillers. Other typical fillers include talc, rice concentrate, cellulose, silica, and magnesium stearate. Vegetarians need to check labels for gelatin, which is made from animals, unless the manufacturer has specified that the capsule is vegetable-based. More and more supplements are available with nonanimal-based capsules and coatings.

Guidelines for Taking Homeopathic Remedies

To be effective, homeopathic remedies need to be taken according to the following specific guidelines.

•*The remedies and dosages in this book are suggestions only. Consult a homeopath or other knowledgeable professional when taking homeopathic remedies.*

•*Homeopathic remedies are available most commonly as tinctures, sugar pills that have been infused with the remedy, granules, or creams.*

•*Before you take a homeopathic remedy, avoid putting anything into your mouth for at least 10 minutes. This includes food, beverages, gum, toothpaste, tobacco smoke, and mouthwash.*

•*If you are taking prescription medications, consult with your physician before you take a homeopathic remedy. Over-the-counter drugs such as aspirin, laxatives, and ibuprofen should be avoided when taking homeopathic remedies.*

•*When giving a remedy to a child, dissolve the tincture, powder, granules, or tablet that you have crushed between two spoons in a little water.*

•*A rule of homeopathic treatment is that once a remedy begins to work, stop taking it or reduce the amount you are taking. Homeopathic remedies stimulate the body's natural healing process, so once healing begins it can continue on its own. If, however, the pain returns in a few hours or the next day, restart the remedy at a higher potency. If you do not get relief after a few more doses, you probably need a different remedy.*

•*During a course of homeopathic treatment, avoid coffee (regular and decaffeinated) because it can negate any benefits from the remedy.*

•Always store homeopathic remedies in a cool, dry, and preferably dark place.

•To determine the proper dose for your needs, refer to the Rule of Three dosage guidelines in the sidebar.

RULE OF THREE: DOSAGE GUIDELINES FOR HOMEOPATHIC REMEDIES

A dose is defined as 5 to 10 drops, 2 to 3 tablets, or 15 to 20 granules. The dosage guidelines listed here can be used when specific recommendations are not given for a particular condition.

For **severe** symptoms: Take 1 dose every 30 to 60 minutes for 3 doses. If there is no relief, repeat as needed up to 24 hours until pain improves to moderate or mild.

For **moderate** symptoms: Take 1 dose every 3 hours for 1 day until symptoms improve to mild.

For **mild** symptoms: Take 1 dose every 6 hours. Repeat as needed for up to 10 days.

Where to Buy Your Remedy

Consumers have a wide variety of options when it comes to where to buy remedies and supplements. Health food stores, vitamin stores, natural food stores, mainstream supermarkets, large chain stores, pharmacies, discount stores, independent distributors, mail order, and the Internet all offer herbal and homeopathic remedies and natural supplements. The more options you have, the more confusing it can be to decide which outlet is best. Generally, health food or vitamin stores have a more diverse selection of remedies and supplements than do other sellers. They are also more likely to carry all-natural brands that avoid the use of additives known as excipients. When treating pain, you want the remedy *now*, so you are less likely to make your first purchase through the mail or over the Internet. However, once you've found a remedy that works for you, you may decide to explore mail order and Internet options, as they often offer discounts. Purchasing remedies through the mail or over the Internet is safe if you know exactly what you want and have already seen the product and know the contents, or if the label is fully available for you to inspect in a catalog or on the website. Do not buy supplements over the telephone from solicitors.

The list in Appendix B represents a very small percentage of the companies that supply herbal and homeopathic remedies and supplements. In no way is it an endorsement of any of these firms. The Internet is an excellent source of suppliers. Search words such as "herbs" or "herbal products" or "supplements" will get you an extensive listing of potential suppliers.

Supplies relating to the mind-body and energy therapies discussed in this book are also provided here, including suppliers of meditation and guided imagery tapes for pain and stress reduction, and magnets. Check your local libraries for audiotapes, where you can borrow them for free.

Glossary

Acetaminophen. An analgesic (painkilling) drug that also reduces fever but is not effective against inflammation. Tylenol is one of the most commonly used acetaminophen products on the market.

Acute. Something that is nonchronic and short in duration. When referring to an illness, one that lasts for no longer than one to two weeks.

Autoimmune disease. A condition in which the body's immune system attacks its own healthy cells.

Ayurveda. The ancient traditional medical system of India that incorporates herbs, meditation, diet, and other natural therapies.

Cartilage. The strong, flexible tissue that supports the bones and joints and makes up some structures, such as the nose and ears.

Chi. In Chinese medicine, the concept alternately known as the vital force, the universal life force, or vital energy. Ideally it flows unhindered throughout the body and is regulated by yin and yang, which govern all things in the universe.

Chronic. Something that is long-term and persistent. When referring to an illness, one that lasts months or years and often requires treatment.

Compress. A piece of soft material formed into a pad that is then soaked in a hot or cold liquid and applied to an external body part.

Decoction. A very strong tea, made from the bark, wood, twigs, or other hard parts of a plant.

Double-blind study. A study in which neither the researcher nor the subject knows when the active substance or the placebo is being used.

Endorphins. A type of chemical compound produced by the body that has pain-relieving properties.

Enteric coating. A special coating applied to a tablet or capsule that prevents it from dissolving in the stomach and thus ensures that it reaches the intestinal tract.

Enzyme. A protein that speeds up certain processes in the body.

Episiotomy. An incision made into the tissues surrounding the opening of the vagina (called the perineum) to make it easier for the infant to come through the birth passage. An episiotomy helps avoid tearing of adjacent tissue during birth.

Extract. The concentrated essence of an herb, which can be provided in a tablet, tincture, powder, or other form of an herb. Extracts usually contain a standardized amount of the active ingredient(s).

Facet joint. A joint formed by the bony protrusions of two adjacent vertebrae.

Herb. A plant or part of a plant that has medicinal value and/or can be used as flavoring in food.

Herniated disk. A condition in which part of the jellylike center of a disk in the spine protrudes through the outer disk wall into the spinal column, pressing against nerves and causing pain.

Hormones. Chemicals produced by the body's glands that have a tremendous effect on the body. They are responsible for tissue repair, growth, reproduction, blood pressure, and how the body responds to stress.

Ibuprofen. An anti-inflammatory drug (e.g., Advil) used to treat painful, inflammatory conditions such as arthritis and menstrual cramps.

Infusion. An herbal remedy that is similar to a tea except more herb is used and it is allowed to steep longer, producing a more potent remedy.

Lumbosacral area. The region on the lower back where the lumbar vertebrae meet the sacrum.

Melatonin. A hormone, produced by the pineal gland, that regulates the body's circadian rhythm (the sleep/awake cycle), influences the cardiovascular and reproductive systems, and affects the immune system.

Neurotransmitter. Any one of many chemicals in the body that transmit messages among the nerve cells.

NSAID. Nonsteroidal anti-inflammatory drug; a drug that reduces inflammation and pain by blocking the production of substances called prostaglandins.

OTC. Over-the-counter. A drug that can be purchased without a doctor's prescription.

pH. A measure of the acidity or alkalinity (baseness) of a substance. The scale ranges from 0 (most acidic) to 14 (most alkaline); 7 is the neutral measure.

Pineal gland. A pea-size gland located deep within the brain that produces the hormone melatonin.

Placebo. A substance often used in scientific studies in which comparisons are made between an active substance and a nonactive (placebo) one. A placebo has no medicinal value but looks like the active ingredient.

Prostaglandins. Hormonelike substances found throughout the body that are involved in numerous processes, including pain.

Reye's syndrome. A rare disorder that occurs during childhood and is apparently caused by aspirin given to children 15 years and younger.

Serotonin. A neurotransmitter that is involved in neurological functions, such as depression, pain, memory, and sleep.

Standardized extract. A concentrated form of an herb that is guaranteed to contain a standardized amount of active ingredients. Standardized forms are not available for all herbs.

Tincture. A liquid form of an herb made by soaking the desired part in water and alcohol.

Vertebrae. The bones that make up the spinal column.

Yin and yang. In Chinese philosophy, the two opposing forces in the universe that are found in all things. Good health depends on the balance of yin and yang, which is demonstrated by the unhindered flow of chi.

Bibliography and Suggested Reading

Alman, Brian M. *Self-Hypnosis: The Complete Manual*. New York: Brunner/Mazel, 1992.

Barnett, Robert A. *Tonics*. New York: Harper Collins, 1997.

Beinfield, H., and E. Korngold. *Between Heaven and Earth: A Guide to Chinese Medicine*. New York: Ballantine, 1991.

Bensky, Dan, and Randall Barolet. *Chinese Herbal Medicine: Formulas & Strategies*. Seattle, WA: Eastland Press, 1990.

Benson, Herbert. *Beyond the Relaxation Response*. New York: Time Books, 1984.

———. *Your Maximum Mind*. New York: Time Books, 1987.

Brand, Paul, and Philip Yancey. *Pain. The Gift Nobody Wants*. New York: HarperCollins, 1993.

Caudill, Margaret A. *Managing Pain Before It Manages You*. New York: Guilford Press, 1995.

Cousins, Norman. *Anatomy of an Illness as Perceived by the Patient*. New York: Norton, 1979.

Duke, James A. *The Green Pharmacy: New Discoveries in Herbal Remedies for Common Diseases and Conditions from the World's Foremost Authority on Healing Herbs.* Emmaus, PA: Rodale Press, 1997.

Foster, Steven. *An Illustrated Guide. 101 Medicinal Herbs.* Fayetteville, AR: Interweave Press, 1998.

Fung, Fung and John Fung. *Sixty Years in Search of Cures. An Herbalist's Success with Chinese Herbs.* Dublin, CA: Get Well Foundation, 1994.

Goleman, Daniel, and Joel Gurin. *Mind Body Medicine.* New York: Consumers Union of United States, 1993.

Graedon, Teresa, and Joe Graedon. *Dangerous Drug Interactions. How To Protect Yourself from Harmful Drug/ Drug, Drug/Food, Drug/Vitamin Combinations.* New York: St. Martins, 1999.

Griffith, H. Winter. *Vitamins, Herbs, Minerals & Supplements.* Tucson, AZ: Fisher Books, 1998.

Grinspoon, Lester, and James Bakalar. *Marijuana: The Forbidden Medicine.* New Haven, CT: Yale University Press, 1997. Available through 1-800-YUP-READ.

Grossingher, Richard. *Homeopathy. An Introduction for Skeptics and Beginners.* Berkeley: North Atlantic Books, 1993.

Harrar, Sari, and Sara Altshul O'Donnell. *Women's Book of Healing Herbs.* Emmaus, PA: Rodale Press, 1999.

Hilgad, Ernest. *Hypnosis: In the Relief of Pain.* New York: Brunner/Mazel, 1994.

Jacob, Stanley, et. al. *The Miracle of MSM: The Natural Solution for Pain.* New York: Penguin, 1999.

Jonas, Wayne B., and Jennifer Jacobs. *Healing with Homeopathy*. New York: Warner Books, 1996.

Kabat-Zinn, Jon. *Full Catastrophe Living: Using the Wisdom of Your Body and Mind to Face Stress, Pain and Illness*. New York: Delacorte, 1991.

————. *Wherever You Go, There You Are: Mindfulness Meditation in Everyday Life*. New York: Hyperion, 1994.

Mindell, Earl. *Dr. Earl Mindell's What You Should Know About Herbs for Your Health*. New Canaan, CT: Keats Publishing, 1996.

Mitchell, Deborah. *MSM. The Natural Pain Relief Remedy*. New York: Avon, 1999.

Murray, Michael T. *The Healing Power of Herbs*. Rocklin, CA: Prima Publishing, 1995.

Naparstek, Belleruth. *Staying Well with Guided Imagery*. New York: Warner Books, 1994

Peirce, Andrea. *The American Pharmaceutical Association. Practical Guide to Natural Medicine*. New York: William Morrow, 1999.

Reid, D. *A Handbook of Chinese Healing Herbs*. Boston: Shambhala Publications, 1995.

Rossman, Martin L. *Healing Yourself: A Step-by-Step Program for Better Health Through Imagery*. New York: Walker & Co., 1987.

Samuels, Michael. *Healing with the Mind's Eye*. New York: Summit Books, 1990.

Siegel, Bernie S. *Love, Medicine and Miracles: Lessons Learned about Self-Healing from a Surgeon's Experi-*

ence with Exceptional Patients. Boston: G. K. Hall, 1988.

————. *Peace, Love & Healing: Bodymind Communication and the Path to Self-Healing*. New York: Harper & Row, 1989.

Theodosakis, Jason. *The Arthritis Cure: The Medical Miracle That Can Halt, Reverse, and May Even Cure Osteoarthritis*. New York: St. Martin's Press, 1997.

Tierra, Lesley. *The Herbs of Life*. Freedom, CA: Crossing Press, 1992.

Tierra, Michael. *Biomagnetics and Herbal Therapy*. Twin Lakes, WI: Lotus Press, 1997.

Tyler, V. *The Honest Herbal*, 3d ed. New York: Haworth Press, 1993.

Ullman, R., and J. Reichenberg-Ullman. *The Patient's Guide to Homeopathic Medicine*. Edmonds, WA: Picnic Point Press, 1995.

Webb, Marcus. *The Herbal Companion*. Allentown, PA: People's Medical Society, 1997.

Weil, Andrew. *From Chocolate to Morphine: Everything You Need to Know about Mind-Altering Drugs*. Boston: Houghton Mifflin, 1993.

Wiseman, Nigel, and Andrew Ellis. *Fundamentals of Chinese Medicine*. Brookline, MA: Paradigm Publications, 1995.

Yates, John. *The Complete Book of Self-Hypnosis*. Chicago: Nelson-Hall, 1984.

Zimmer, L., and J. P. Morgan. *Marijuana Myth, Marijuana Facts: A Review of the Scientific Evidence*. New York: Lindesmith Center, 1997.

Zimmerman, Bill, Rick Bayer, and Nancy Crumpacker. *Is Marijuana the Right Medicine for You?* New Canaan, CT: Keats Publishing, 1998.

APPENDIX A

Organizations of Interest

Academy for Guided Imagery
PO Box 2070
Mill Valley, CA 94942
800-726-2070
www.interactiveimagery.com

American Botanical Council
PO Box 201660
Austin, TX 78720
512-331-8868
E-mail: abc@herbalgram.org
www.herbalgram.org

The American Association of Oriental Medicine
433 Front Street
Catasauqua, PA 18032
610-266-1433
E-mail: aaom1@aol.com
www.aaom.org

American Chronic Pain Association
PO Box 850
Rocklin, CA 95677
916-632-0922
www.theacpa.org

American Herbalist Guild
PO Box 70
Roosevelt, UT 84066
435-722-8434
E-mail: ahgoffice@earthlink.net
www.earthlink.net

American Society of Clinical Hypnosis
2200 East Devon Avenue, Suite 291
Des Plaines, IL 60018

Biofeedback Certification Institute of America
10200 West 44th Avenue, Suite 304
Wheatridge, CO 80033
Referrals to biofeedback practitioners

Herb Research Foundation
1007 Pearl Street, Suite 200
Boulder, CO 80302
303-449-2265
E-mail: info@herbs.org
www.herbs.org

Homeopathic Educational Services
2124 Kittredge Street
Berkeley, CA 94704
510-649-0294
800-359-9051
www.homeopathic.com

Marijuana Websites:
Alliance for Cannabis Therapeutics:
www.marijuana-as-medicine.org/alliance.htm
Who Supports Access to Medical Marijuana?:
www.marijuana-as-medicine.org/support.html

National Center for Homeopathy
801 N Fairfax, Suite 306
Alexandria, VA 22314
703-548-7790
Clearinghouse for information about homeopathy; a
monthly newsletter; network of study groups around
the country
www.homeopathic.org

National Chronic Pain Outreach Association
7979 Old Georgetown Road, Suite 100
Bethesda, MD 20814-2429
301-652-4948

Stress Reduction Clinic
University of Massachusetts Medical Center
Worcester, MA 01655
508-856-1616

Mail-Order and Internet Sources

Herbs and Homeopathic Remedies

Avena Botanicals
219 Mill Street
Rockport, ME 04856
Tinctures, bulk herbs, and books
www.avenaherbs.com

Boericke & Tafel, Inc.
Santa Rosa, CA 95407
505-473-1717
Homeopathic remedies

East Earth Trade Winds
PO Box 493151
Redding, CA 96049-3151
800-258-6878
Catalog, Chinese tonic formulas and bulk Chinese
herbs
www.eastearthtrade.com

Gaia Herbs
108 Island Ford Road
Brevard, NC 28712
828-884-4242
Tinctures, including Chinese and Ayurvedic

Hadas Natural Products
PO Box 48059
Atlanta, GA 30362
800-99-HADAS
Homeopathic remedies

Homeopathic Overnight
4111 Simon Road
Youngstown, OH 44512
800-ARNICA30

Institute Herb Company
1190 Northeast 125th Street
N Miami, FL 33161
305-899-8704
Catalog; bulk Chinese and Western herbs and tonic
formulas

Mountain Herbals
7 Langdon Street
Montpelier, VT 05602-2908
Write for catalog; dried herbs, tinctures, and custom
formulas

St. John's Herb Garden
PO Box 70
Bowie, MD 20720
Herb plants, dried herbs, teas, Chinese herbs

Tea Garden Herbal Emporium
903 Colorado Avenue, Suite 120
Santa Monica, CA 90401
800-288-HERB
Catalog; Chinese tonic formulas and bulk herbs

Audiotapes

Health Journeys
Time Warner AudioBooks
9229 Sunset Boulevard
Los Angeles, CA 90069
Guided imagery audiotapes

Meditations for Everyday Living, by Bernie Siegel, M.D.
1302 Chapel Street
New Haven, CT 06511
203-865-8392

The Present Moment: A Retreat on the Practice of Mindfulness, by Thich Nhat Hanh
Sounds True
800-333-9185
Audiocassettes on meditation

Source Cassette Learning System
945 Evelyn Street
Menlo Park, CA 94025
415-328-7171
Tapes for pain relief, surgery preparation, and healing

Magnet Therapy

East West School of Herbalism
Box 712
Santa Cruz, CA 95061
800-717-5010
www.cruzio.com/~eastwest
Ask for catalog of magnets, magnet supplies; also offers the East West Herbal Correspondence Course and seminars by Dr. Michael Tierra

Internatural
33719 116th Street
Twin Lakes, WI 53181
800-643-4221 (orders)
www.netmart.com/internatural
Suppliers of herbs, magnets, supplements, and other alternative health items

Norso Biomagnetics
4105 Starboard Court
Raleigh, NC 27613
800-480-8601
Suppliers of magnetic pads, wraps, etc.
www.norso.com

Space Age Bio-magnetic Products
27126B Paseo Espada, Suite 701
San Juan Capistrano, CA 92675
714-248-5212
800-861-0513
Biomagnetic products
www.space-age.com/spaceage